FAST YOURSELF

USING **FASTING** AND **LOW-CARB EATING**

TO **LOSE WEIGHT** AND **FEEL GREAT**

EMMA VAN CARLEN

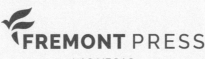

FREMONT PRESS

LAS VEGAS

First published in 2025 by Fremont Press
Copyright © 2025 Emma Van Carlen

ISBN-13: 978-1628605-11-2

Cover design by Kat Lannom
Cover photo by Martin Van Carlen
Interior design and illustrations by Elita San Juan and Crizalie Olimpo

Printed in the USA
POD 0125

Disclaimer

The information included in this book is for educational purposes only. It is not intended or implied to be a substitute for professional medical advice. The reader should always consult their healthcare provider to determine the appropriateness of the information for their own situation or if they have any questions regarding a medical condition or treatment plan. Reading the information in this book does not constitute a physician-patient relationship. This book details the author's personal experiences with and opinions about fasting, diet, and weight loss. The author is not a healthcare provider.

The author and publisher are providing this book and its contents on an "as is" basis and make no representations or warranties of any kind with respect to this book or its contents. The author and publisher disclaim all such representations and warranties, including, for example, warranties of merchantability and healthcare for a particular purpose. In addition, the author and publisher do not represent or warrant that the information accessible via this book is accurate, complete, or current.

The statements in this book have not been evaluated by the Food and Drug Administration. The products or supplements in this book are not intended to diagnose, treat, cure, or prevent any disease. The authors and publisher expressly disclaim responsibility for any adverse effects that may result from the use or application of the information contained in this book.

Please consult with your own physician or healthcare specialist regarding the suggestions and recommendations made in this book.

Neither the author or publisher, nor any authors, contributors, or other representatives, will be liable for damages arising out of or in connection with the use of this book. This is a comprehensive limitation of liability that applies to all damages of any kind, including (without limitation) compensatory; direct, indirect or consequential damages; loss of data, income, or profit; loss of or damage to property; and claims of third parties.

This book is not intended as a substitute for consultation with a licensed healthcare practitioner, such as your physician. Before you begin any healthcare program or change your lifestyle in any way, you should consult your physician or another licensed healthcare practitioner to ensure that you are in good health and that the examples contained in this book will not harm you.

This book provides content related to physical and/or mental health issues. As such, use of this book implies your acceptance of this disclaimer.

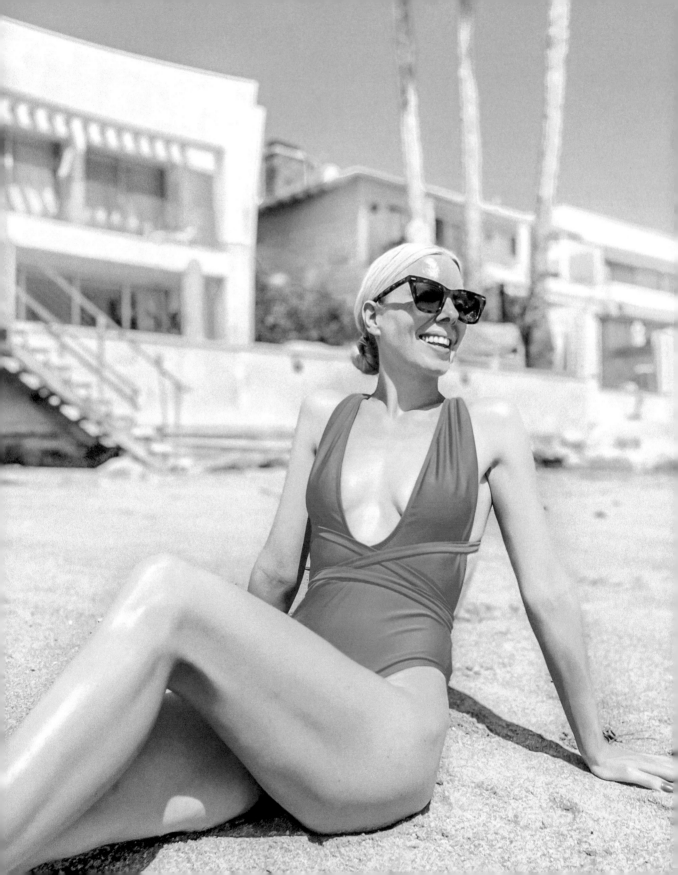

CONTENTS

INTRODUCTION

I've struggled with my weight my whole adult life, and I've tried pretty much all the diets under the sun, but every time I tried a new diet to lose weight and get healthy, I failed.

I simply never understood diets and wasn't able to make them work for me. I was in a constant yo-yo cycle for years, forever gaining more weight and more inflammation, and it was catastrophic for both my physical and my mental health.

So when I was getting ready for my wedding in 2019, I just knew something had to change. Something switched in me at that time, and I was able to lose 30 pounds in the year leading up to my wedding. I felt the most amazing I had ever felt in my body.

Reaching my goal weight has been such an incredible, liberating feeling, and the best part is that I've been able to maintain the weight loss. I now feel free and beautiful in my body, and I no longer struggle with negative body image issues.

I wanted to write this book to share how discovering fasting completely changed my life. I hope to help other people who are in the same place that I was—bloated, unhappy, struggling with their weight, and have tried 100 different diets without any of them working. I know firsthand just how frustrating and distressing that can be. After reaching my goal weight, resolving my hormonal issues, and finally cracking the code to losing weight and keeping it off, I knew I had to share this knowledge with other people.

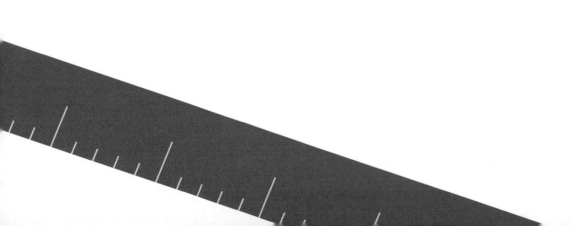

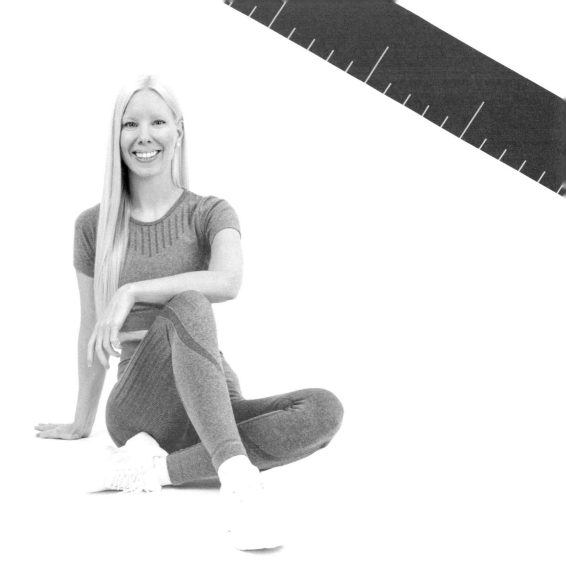

My Story

I wasn't always overweight. In fact, I was always a skinny kid growing up, and food didn't interest me much. I could easily eat when I was hungry and not eat when I wasn't. But somewhere along the way, I lost that ability, as a lot of people do.

As a child, I was blissfully protected from diet culture much longer than many young girls seem to be today. I made it all the way to junior high without really thinking much about how I looked. I never spent a significant time in front of the mirror, and I generally dressed in whatever I thought was comfortable before I headed out the door in the mornings.

That all changed when I was around 14 years old. I remember being in the changing room after gym class. As I was pulling up my jeans, one of my friends looked over, pointed at my belly, and said, "Looks like you're getting some rolls there." I can tell you for a fact I was not getting "rolls." I was a slim 14-year-old. Also, isn't your stomach supposed to "roll" when you bend down? Even still, her comment stuck with me, and from that point on, I started my complicated relationship with my body, food, and the mirror.

I spent my teenage years influenced by diet culture and slowly started gaining weight through unhealthy eating habits. As most individuals following a Western way of eating, my diet was full of sugars, refined vegetable oils, and highly processed carbs—a combination that ended up being disastrous for me.

Around that time, I went on my first diet. My friend and I decided to cut out all white bread, sugar, pasta, and other sweet treats. It was really difficult, but at the end of the eight weeks, my body had gotten used to having less sugar. My first taste of cake or chocolate after this period was sickeningly sweet. However, neither of us lost any significant amount of weight because our carb and sugar intake were still very high. We had swapped our white bread for brown bread, white pasta for whole grain, and refined sugar for copious amounts of dried fruit (which is still very high in sugar). If I knew then what I know now about the relationship between carbohydrates, insulin, and weight gain, I could have avoided years of yo-yo dieting.

~~white bread~~
~~sugar~~
~~pasta~~
~~sweets~~

THE FRESHMAN FIFTEEN

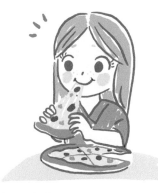

When I started university, I quickly realized why the phrase "freshman fifteen" exists. I was living my best life, enjoying living on my own for the first time and eating all the food, candy, and late-night takeout a girl could muster. But the more I was enjoying myself, the more my waistline was expanding. I tried to mitigate this with periods of calorie restriction and intense cardio at the gym, but I could only sustain this for a week or two before I would go back to eating junk again. This back-and-forth dieting made me miserable, and it certainly didn't make me maintain any meaningful weight loss. In fact, with each passing semester, I was heavier and more unhealthy than the one before.

Because of the strain of the intense cardio sessions and the intense hunger from calorie restriction, I also developed a bit of a binge-eating habit. Whenever I felt like I couldn't handle my restrictive diet anymore, I would raid the cupboards and go to the corner store to buy everything in sight; I'd eat most of it in one sitting. In the end, I felt that I had lost control with food, and I was often finding myself compulsively overeating and feeling bad about myself as a result. I was bloated, heavier than ever, and I had so much inflammation in my body that I had developed adult-onset cystic acne. I had never struggled with acne in my teenage years, but during this time, my jaw and neck were full of red, painful cysts. Consequently, I took strong medications and antibiotics for years as I tried (unsuccessfully) to deal with it. Consuming all that high-carb, processed food had caused my body to become inflamed and pushed my hormonal balance out of sync.

It was around this time that I discovered fasting. I had watched a documentary about the health and weight-loss benefits of fasting two days a week, so I decided to give it a go. Without really doing any further research, I threw caution to the wind and started a three-day fast. By the end of Day 2, I felt so miserable, hungry, nauseated, and headachy that I couldn't take it anymore, and I ended the fast early. I thought maybe fasting wasn't for me, so I went back to cardio and calorie counting and continued to gain more and more weight as a result.

After about another year of feeling miserable and growing ever more tired of my hormonal issues, I did more research into fasting. I read books and joined online fasting support groups. Armed with my newfound knowledge, I was able to complete a couple of forty-eight-hour fasts with success. I felt euphoric! I felt as if I had cracked the code to life. I was walking around town, not having eaten anything for more than twenty-four hours, and running on my own stored body fat without feeling much hunger at all. Did no one else know this was possible? I felt like I had discovered the secret to effortless weight loss, and I finally started to feel healthier and less inflamed.

Then life happened again. I moved to Los Angeles and started working toward my master's degree. I loved the sun and the beach, and I was doing well academically, but being away from home was a lot for me to take. While my grades were soaring, my mental health was plummeting. I found myself once again in the throes of binge eating, calorie restriction, and excessive cardio. And, of course, I gained weight quickly.

I tried to shrug it off. I thought maybe this was just my new, more mature body, and I needed to find a way to accept it for what it was. I wasn't 16 anymore, so I couldn't possibly expect to have the same body that I had back then. I leaned into body positivity and tried to convince myself that my physical form didn't matter, but deep down inside, I knew I was lying to myself. Every time I saw a picture of myself, I felt mortified. I felt as though the person staring back at me from the photo was not the same person I was inside. It wasn't really me. It was someone who was sad and bloated and struggled to find balance in her life.

And then I got engaged. My boyfriend of ten years proposed to me on a trip around the Grand Canyon. I was ecstatic, but I was also terrified. How was I going to get married feeling like this? I knew I needed to do something about my weight and health, and I knew the only way to do so was fasting.

SHEDDING FOR THE WEDDING

I decided to throw myself further into fasting research with a determination to do it right this time. I switched to a ketogenic diet and started a one meal a day (OMAD) schedule. The impending wedding day gave me more motivation and determination than I'd had in previous attempts, and because I knew from experience that fasting worked, I was able to relax more and trust the process. I quickly felt better and more energetic, and I could make healthier food choices easily. In the first month of OMAD, I lost 12 pounds. After a month of OMAD, I was ready to try more extended fasts.

Trying extended fasts was empowering. I experienced some hunger, but it wasn't too bad. In fact, I was surprised by the amount of energy I had when I went for my daily one-hour walks. On day four of my fast, I even went for a run. It felt magical to literally be running on empty. I was finally discovering what the human body was capable of and designed to do—to use our body fat to supply us with energy.

Doing extended fasting was enlightening in several ways. I quickly realized that although some of the physical symptoms, like hunger, were challenging at times, but it was my mind that was my biggest obstacle. I frequently had an inner dialogue running about whether I should quit or keep going and whether I should go back to calorie counting or try a different, less challenging, fasting schedule instead.

Because overcoming negative thoughts was my biggest challenge, I created a list of reasons why I was doing my fast as well as a list of all of the excuses I could think of for breaking my fast. I was effectively trying to outsmart my mind before it had a chance to trick me. I read them every day and every time I felt like breaking my fast. The lists reminded me why I was fasting and of all the excuses I could make that weren't appropriate reasons for breaking my fast; they really kept me going in those difficult moments. (I always recommend that my clients create these lists for themselves.)

Fasting had completely changed my life by this point. My inflammation went down, I was less bloated, I had more energy, and I was finally losing weight. On top of those things, fasting had done what years of strong medications hadn't been able to do: It had cleared up my cystic acne. I saw the biggest results when I combined fasting with a strict keto diet.

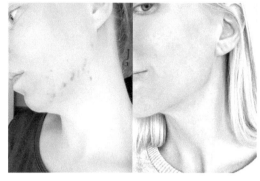

By the time of my bachelorette party, I was at my goal weight and felt better than ever. I felt confident in my body, and my mind was locked in. I was so committed that on my bachelorette party weekend, I stuck 100 percent to a ketogenic diet because I knew I didn't want to undo all the hard work and all the progress I had made. I still had a keto-friendly drink and thoroughly enjoyed myself with my girls. It was such an empowering and liberating feeling knowing that I could enjoy all of these things without compromising my health and body goals.

On my wedding day, I was still at my goal weight, and I felt the most beautiful I had ever felt. I told myself that my wedding was a free-for-all, and I planned to get back to my healthy eating habits the day after. But that's where it all went wrong.

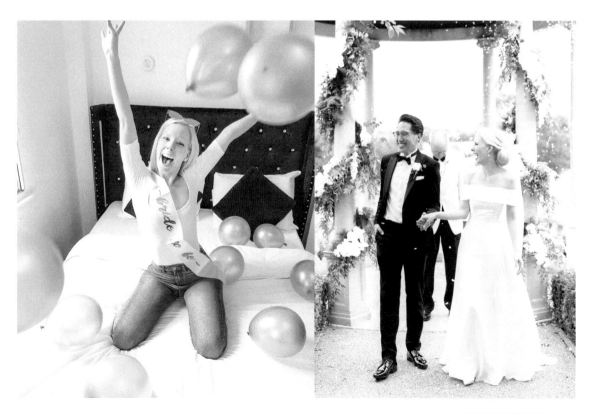

I GAINED IT ALL BACK

After the wedding, it was as if a switch had flipped in my brain. I felt like I was physically and mentally unable to get back to all the things that had worked so well for me in the past. I struggled with staying on a keto diet, and I even struggled with the shortest fasts. Most days, I didn't even make it sixteen hours. I completely lost touch with my calm and centered mindset, and I proceeded to eat anything and everything in sight. I had discovered the true secret to weight loss, so why was I gaining it all back?

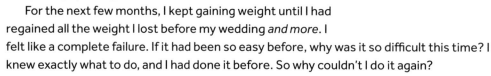

In the space of a week, I regained 15 pounds. I was swollen, bloated, and miserable, and I didn't like the person staring back at me from the mirror. I was crying every day because I felt so out of control. I felt as if I had lost myself, and I was completely spiraling.

For the next few months, I kept gaining weight until I had regained all the weight I lost before my wedding *and more*. I felt like a complete failure. If it had been so easy before, why was it so difficult this time? I knew exactly what to do, and I had done it before. So why couldn't I do it again?

FIGURING OUT WHAT WORKED FOR ME

Ultimately, the key to my success was being so tired of my own ways that there was no other way out but to change. That's not to say the road was easy. I had been tired of my own behavior and excuses many times before, but perhaps I hadn't been tired *enough* to produce lasting change.

Many times, I had thought that I could do intermittent fasting through the week and then allow myself to have a cheat meal on the weekend. However, doing that would lead to a cheat weekend, which would then turn into a cheat week, and before I knew it, I was completely out of control. Even the times when I was able to keep my unhealthy eating to just one day, I gained so much weight because of excess inflammation and water weight that I felt extremely uncomfortable. In addition, it took me a full week of hard work to get back to the weight I had been before the cheat day. Instead of using that week to make further progress, I had to use that whole week just to get back to where I had been a week before.

So when I made my final, lasting change, the first thing I did was cut out "cheat days." I knew that if I wanted to be serious and get the results I desired, I needed to be consistent and committed. No excuses.

FINALLY CRACKING THE CODE: THE PRINCIPLES OF FASTING

What I liked about getting back into my journey this time around was that I'd already done it all once before. I had already lost 30 pounds using these exact methods, so I knew I had the capacity to do it again. I no longer had the mental block of being unable to see myself achieving my goals. Before I lost the weight the first time around, I thought maybe losing weight wasn't possible for me or that I couldn't achieve the body I imagined. But since I'd been able to do it once before and had felt amazing on my wedding day, I knew it was achievable, and I had confidence that I could do it one more time.

But having the tools is one thing—using them is another.

I again started with a month of keto OMAD. By the end of the month, I had some great results. I lost 8 pounds, which I was ecstatic about. After that, despite my plan, I had some cheat meals, which derailed me a bit, but I was able to get back on track relatively quickly.

That's when I started to get into extended fasting a bit more. I did a couple of four-day fasts, a five-day fast, and a seven-day fast. In between, I was eating either one or two meals a day. And I was eating healthy and delicious keto foods. These patterns really worked for me because I was able to fast around my social schedule. I could eat dinner with my husband in the evenings on my OMAD schedule, and I made sure to schedule my extended fasts for days when I didn't have any big social obligations. It's important to note that extended fasting should always be approached with caution, and you especially need to take care to have a safe refeed (more on this in Chapter 12).

Eating keto was also a lot smoother this time because I had figured out which types of food I liked and which types of meals were easy and accessible for me. I already had my favorites, and I kept going back to them.

It took me a couple of months of moderately slow progress before I decided to go on my longest fast ever, which ended up being eighteen days. I had never done such a long fast before. Seven days had been my max. I had a personal goal of completing a full three-week fast—twenty-one days—so that's what I set out to do. I had my electrolytes, my mindset was strong, and I was ready to give it my all.

The first few days were pretty difficult, but then I built some momentum and it got easier. Sure, I experienced some hunger and had some headaches and nausea, but nothing I couldn't handle. By day seven, I had already lost 10 pounds, and that really motivated me to keep going. In the second week, I experienced side effects that were a bit more uncomfortable, but hunger wasn't really an issue. The most uncomfortable side effect was the absence of the social aspect of eating with others. I had asked my husband to eat in a separate room to avoid triggering me. I was locked into my goal, and I wasn't going to let anything derail me.

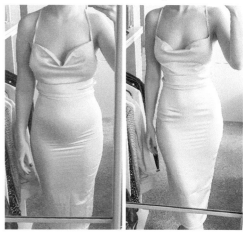

Through fasting, and extended fasting in particular, I realized how much time we spend eating food, thinking about eating food, or planning our next meal. Having this realization prompted me to explore other ways to keep myself occupied and mentally and emotionally fulfilled. Instead of seeing food as my main source of enjoyment, I filled my time with socializing, walks, and other relaxing activities.

By the third week, I was ready to throw in the towel. Not physically—my body was doing fine—but mentally I was struggling with self-sabotage. I was sailing through the days, and by day eighteen, I had convinced myself that because it was so easy for me to fast, I knew I was going to make it to twenty-one days. Any doubts I previously had regarding whether I was going to make it were completely gone. I had made it eighteen days, and I felt great, so making it another three days was going to be a piece of cake. In thinking that, I convinced myself that I didn't need to prove anything. So if I felt too bored or if I missed food too much, it was perfectly fine for me to break my fast. Unfortunately, I was not strong enough to resist these powerful thoughts, and on day eighteen, I broke my fast.

I was really proud of myself for making it eighteen days, and I was calm and centered enough to break my fast slowly before moving into a long and careful refeed during which I kept my carbs extremely low to avoid overwhelming my system. However, I was disappointed that I didn't make it the full twenty-one days. I wish I had pushed myself past those mental barriers to make it the full three weeks, as was my original plan. The eighteen-day fast was a huge learning experience for me, and I lost 17 pounds in the process.

Note: Please remember that long extended fasts such as this one are not recommended for beginners, and you should always make sure you have your doctor's approval and supervision, if necessary.

After a few more bumps in the road, I finally reached my goal weight again, and I felt absolutely amazing. Since then, I have not let self-sabotage get in the way, and I am still at my goal today.

Cracking the code and discovering the principles to fasting for weight loss felt like winning the lottery. After struggling with my weight my whole adulthood, I feel like I have a new lease on life. I'm able to enjoy getting dressed in the morning and clothes shopping, and I love looking at myself in the mirror. I used to hate going to the beach because I didn't

like how I looked and felt in a swimsuit. But now I love going to the beach, and I look forward to all the pictures that we take at every new location because I feel so good in my body. I've also improved my health immensely: I've healed my cystic acne, and I no longer struggle with inflammation. I'm so much calmer and happier in my mind.

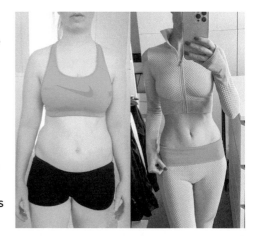

That's what I want for you. If I can do it, you can too. So if you're in a doubt about whether losing the weight and getting to grips with your unhealthy eating habits is going to be worth it, let me tell you: It is 100 percent worth it, and you will not regret this journey.

Why I Wrote This Book

I am a Harvard-trained health advocate and writer, and working with people and helping people has always been something I've been passionate about. I have an educational background in both psychology and counseling, with a master of arts in psychology, a master of communication management, and a diploma in counseling. I base a lot of my teachings and methods on this training. My work as a health educator and fasting and accountability coach allows me to help thousands of people improve their health, lose weight, and feel amazing in their bodies every year.

Through my work, I know just how big of an impact fasting can have, and I am always on a mission to find ways to reach more people and transform more lives. Writing this book was the perfect avenue for that. This book contains all the knowledge, insights, and lessons I've learned through my own health and weight-loss journey, as well as from working with thousands of clients all over the world.

Losing weight doesn't have to involve spending hours at the gym, feeling hungry constantly, and restricting yourself with hard-to-manage diets. I've discovered that there is a better way. Through this book, I will demystify the weight-loss process and give you a simple, practical, and sustainable way to lose weight and improve health that actually works.

There are a few things I hope you to take away from this book:

- **Why conventional diets fail:** Most traditional diets focus on cutting calories and working out, but they all fail to understand the underlying hormonal imbalances that cause weight gain in the first place. I will teach you why traditional diets don't work and why it's not your fault that you're gaining weight.

- **How people have fasted throughout history and why it's a healthy approach:** Fasting is nothing new. In fact, it's been practiced for thousands of years for health, weight loss, and spiritual reasons. I'll tell you about the history of fasting and why it's the most natural thing you can do for your body.

- **What the hormonal foundations of weight gain and insulin resistance are:** You need to understand that weight gain is not just about calories in versus calories out. Instead, it's about hormones—particularly insulin. I'll go through the main hormonal drivers behind your weight gain and how you can manipulate and balance those hormones to start losing weight effectively.

- **How to lose weight through fasting—without hitting the gym:** I'll give you a step-by-step guide for starting fasting, explain the fasting schedule options, and show you how to choose which fasting schedule fits you the best. I'll give you practical guidelines on how to fast correctly and how to stay motivated when it gets tough.

- **How to change your diet to lose weight effortlessly:** Losing weight isn't just about how much you eat; it's also about what you eat. I'll explain how to change your diet to balance your hormones and lose weight without restricting.

- **How to keep weight off in the long run by listening to your body and practicing mindful eating:** I'll cover how to maintain your weight through the principles of mindful eating once you've reached your goal weight so that you can discover food freedom and never have to go on a diet again.

This book is more than just a simple guide to fasting. It provides a complete foundation for you to understand how your body works and how you can take control of your weight once and for all. By the end of this book, you'll have the tools that you need to finally reach your goal weight and maintain it for the rest of your life.

Is There Anyone Who Shouldn't Be Fasting?

Fasting is a great way to improve your health and lose weight, but it's not for everyone. The following people should not be fasting:

- **Anyone under 18:** If you're younger than 18, you should not be fasting because your body is still developing. Your body requires all the nutrients it can get to grow and develop appropriately, which means fasting isn't safe for you.

- **Anyone with an eating disorder:** If you have an eating disorder, fasting is not for you. A lot of people confuse fasting with an eating disorder, but this couldn't be further from the truth. Fasting is a conscious health practice, whereas an eating disorder is a complex mental health condition. If you've been diagnosed with an eating disorder, fasting could potentially make any underlying issues with food and body image worse.

- **People who are underweight:** If you're underweight, or if you're close to being underweight, you shouldn't be fasting. Fasting will cause you to lose a lot of weight quickly, so if you're already at a low weight, fasting could put you in a dangerous health situation.

- **Anyone who's pregnant or breastfeeding:** Fasting while pregnant is not recommended. This is because when you're pregnant, your body needs as many nutrients as possible to feed the growing baby and provide energy for you. After delivery—and after finishing breastfeeding, if you choose to do it—you can resume fasting to shed any extra baby weight.

- **People with chronic diseases or underlying health conditions:** Fasting can do wonders to improve various health conditions including obesity, type 2 diabetes, and even some cancers. But because each of these conditions requires complex medical treatment, it's important that you always consult a doctor before attempting to incorporate any fasting into your daily routine. This will ensure that fasting is appropriate for your unique situation and allow your doctor to make any appropriate adjustments to medications.

Now that you know my story, let's move on to talking about how fasting works and why it's great for your health. Chapter 1 explores the mechanics behind how fasting is such a powerful weight-loss tool.

1

THE WHAT AND WHY OF FASTING

CHAPTER 1
WHAT IS FASTING?

In its simplest definition, *fasting* means you don't eat any food at all for a specific period of time: a certain number of hours, days, or even weeks, depending on which fasting schedule you choose. Fasting has been practiced for religious, cultural, and health reasons for millennia.

In this chapter, I go over the basics behind how and why fasting works, introduce your body's two fuel systems, explain the role of insulin in weight gain (and weight loss), and tell you how fasting is different from starvation. Finally, I outline the many benefits of fasting that go way beyond just weight loss.

The BASIC MECHANICS of FASTING

The human body stores energy in the form of body fat. When you're fasting, your body shifts its main source of energy from the carbohydrates in the food you eat to your stored body fat.

This metabolic shift, called ketosis, is when your body fat is broken down into ketones to be used for energy when there is no food available.

Ketosis normally starts after a person has gone without eating for twelve to twenty-four hours. The actual amount of time can vary from person to person depending on each individual's metabolism and what diet they're following before the fast.

Fasting helps you develop better metabolic health by improving your insulin sensitivity and lowering your blood sugar levels; it reduces inflammation and can even improve your brain performance. Fasting helps you lose weight easily, and it also reduces your risk of developing type 2 diabetes and other metabolic disorders.

There are many different types of fasting schedules. Some examples are intermittent fasting, where you fast for some portion of each day; alternate-day fasting, where you switch between fasting and eating every other day; and extended fasting, where you fast for a few days in a row. I provide more detail about the various schedules in Chapter 2.

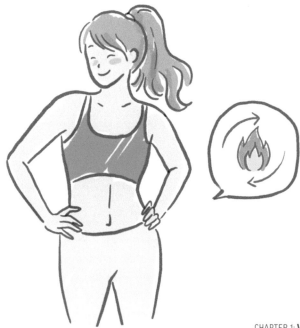

Your Body's Two Energy Systems: Ketosis and Glycolysis

The first step for using fasting to lose weight is to understand the science behind how it works and *why it works*.

Your body runs on two systems—it can either burn carbs for fuel (through a process called *glycolysis*), or it can burn stored body fat for fuel (through *ketosis*), but it can't do both at the same time. Think of it as a hybrid car, which can either run on gasoline (fuel you put in the tank) or electricity (fuel the car has stored). It can't run on both types of fuel at the same time. If you want to lose weight, you need to understand the relationship between these two fuel systems.

GLYCOLYSIS & GLYCOGENESIS

Glycolysis is just a fancy word for how your body breaks down glucose (sugar and carbs) to produce energy. It's the most common way your body makes energy. The easiest way to explain glycolysis is that when you eat carbs, they're broken down into glucose that you either use for energy right away or store in your cells as glycogen for use later. Storing unused glucose is called glycogenesis.

You have some glycogen stores in your liver and muscles, but when those glycogen stores are filled up, any excess glycogen is stored as body fat. The reason many of us struggle with carrying too much weight is that we eat more (carbs) than our bodies need, and all that extra energy is stored as fat to be used on a rainy day. The problem in modern society is that the rainy day never comes. We keep eating and keep storing, and we never allow our bodies to use any of that delicious stored body fat.

The other major downside to relying only on glycolysis as your energy source is that it leads to carb cravings and sugar crashes because you've taught your body it needs carbs to function. So if you rely on glycolysis all of the time, it puts you at a metabolic disadvantage. Instead, you should aim for metabolic flexibility.

KETOSIS

Metabolic flexibility is where ketosis comes in. Ketosis is a metabolic process where your body switches from burning carbs (glucose) for fuel to burning your stored body fat for fuel. The only way ketosis can happen is when your body is shut off from its usual fuel source—carbohydrates.

The best way to put your body into ketosis is through fasting, a low-carbohydrate diet, or a combination of the two. When you fast, your body quickly uses the glycogen stored in your liver and muscles and then starts to look for other sources of energy. When there's no more glycogen in your system, your body starts running on ketones by breaking down stored body fat. This shows how easily your body adapts when there's no food (or no carbs) around.

Fasting is like a gearshift; it switches your body from glycolysis to ketosis—moving you from burning food for fuel to burning body fat for fuel. Once your body gets used to fasting, you become more metabolically flexible, meaning you can effortlessly switch between and tap into both of these energy systems at the drop of a hat.

This metabolic shift from burning glycogen to burning ketones not only helps you lose weight by using your stored body fat but also gives you a steady supply of energy (because you have an almost endless supply of stored body fat). As a result, you don't get the typical energy fluctuations and sugar crashes you normally get from eating a high-carbohydrate diet.

What Is Autophagy?

Fasting also puts your body into autophagy, which is a natural process where your body removes and recycles old and damaged cells and other tissue to produce new, healthy ones. Think of it as your body's spring-cleaning system. The word consists of two parts:

- *auto*, which means *self*
- *phagy*, which means *eat*

So the literal translation of the word *autophagy* is *self-eating*. Your body basically eats itself.

Autophagy is an important process that's necessary to keep your body running smoothly. It's triggered when there's no food or other nutrients coming into your system, which means that fasting is the best way to activate it. Because it gets rid of old and damaged cells and only leaves those that function well, it prevents waste from building inside your cells. This means that autophagy can reduce your risk for developing neurodegenerative disorders like Alzheimer's and Parkinson's diseases. Autophagy also makes it easier for your immune system to recognize threats and keep infections down, and it can reduce your risk for developing cancer because it stops the buildup of defective DNA and other cell parts that can cause cancer to grow.

Autophagy is the reason it's so important to give your digestive system a break from eating; your body can't run properly if you feed it around the clock. When you're constantly eating, you disrupt your body's healing and deep-cleaning processes, and you increase your risk of developing a whole host of diseases and ailments. Frequently activating autophagy in your body can improve your overall health.

Why Fasting Works

Understanding the role of insulin is the most important step in changing your perception of how fat-burning happens. Knowing about insulin also helps you understand why it's almost impossible to lose weight if you keep eating.

One of insulin's most important roles is as a fat-storage hormone. Simply put, when insulin levels are high, you store body fat; when insulin levels are low, you burn body fat.

Insulin is produced in your pancreas and released into your bloodstream every time you eat. The food you eat is converted into glucose (sugar) in your blood, and insulin helps to transport that glucose from your blood into your cells.

After you eat, particularly when you eat food high in carbohydrates, insulin levels increase to help cells take up all the extra glucose from the bloodstream so you can use it as energy. When the amount of glucose is higher than what your body needs right away, insulin also helps store the excess glucose as body fat. This is an important and natural process in your body, and when insulin levels are triggered intermittently, your body can handle it really well. But when you're constantly eating and snacking on high-carb food, your insulin levels are continuously triggered, leading to chronically high insulin levels. That's when you run into problems with weight gain. When your insulin levels stay high over a long period, your body stores fat rather than burns it as fuel, which eventually leads to insulin resistance.

If you become insulin resistant, your cells aren't able to react to insulin in the proper way, meaning they can't pick up all that extra glucose. And because your cells aren't reacting properly to the insulin being released, your pancreas has no choice but to release even greater amounts of insulin into your blood, which results in more fat being stored on your body. These chronically high levels of insulin cause you to gain more and more weight as your body continues to live in a constant state of fat storage. Unless you find a way to decrease your insulin levels, you're effectively blocking your body from burning your body fat.

On top of causing your body to store fat, another effect of high insulin levels is that it can change your normal hunger and appetite control. Insulin affects your hypothalamus, a region in your brain that deals with appetite regulation. When you keep triggering high insulin by constantly eating, you can have more cravings, which results in eating more and gaining more weight because you're trapped in a vicious cycle of hunger, overeating, and fat storage.

By fasting, you break out of this vicious cycle. Fasting lowers your insulin and activates ketosis. Lowering your insulin levels basically tells your body to go from fat-storage mode to fat-burning mode.

You can only lower your insulin levels by not eating at all or by eating less—particularly by eating fewer carbohydrates. When carbohydrates are low, your liver is forced to convert fatty acids into ketones to be used as an alternative source of energy. One of the reasons fasting is so effective for weight loss is because it helps you tap into the metabolic processes that have been interrupted by the constant eating patterns of modern society.

Fasting speeds up the metabolic process by emptying your body's carbohydrate stores quicker. A key benefit of ketosis (other than fat-burning, of course) is that it helps suppress hunger, which is very helpful when you're fasting.

This whole process doesn't just help you lose weight; it also helps to improve your insulin sensitivity, which helps you maintain a healthy weight in the long run and reduces your risk for developing type 2 diabetes and other metabolic disorders. By reducing how often you eat through intermittent fasting, you minimize the number of insulin spikes you get every day, which helps you regulate both your blood sugar and insulin levels.

Following a ketogenic diet is another way to promote ketosis in the body, and because a ketogenic diet mimics the effects of fasting, it will make you lose weight and improve your metabolism. So when you combine fasting with a ketogenic diet, you maximize ketosis, which in turn helps you maximize both the amount of weight you lose and the positive changes to your metabolic health.

Fasting Is Not the Same as Starvation

One of the most common concerns people have when they first hear about fasting is that they'll starve. *Fasting* and starving should never be used interchangeably because they don't mean the same thing at all. Fasting is voluntary and can be used in a controlled way to improve a variety of health conditions and promote weight loss, *whereas* starvation is an involuntary and dangerous condition that can result in organ failure and death. In the following sections, I discuss the differences between fasting and starvation.

FASTING IS VOLUNTARY

First, fasting is voluntary, and starvation is not. In the simplest terms, fasting is a voluntary practice where you choose to abstain from food for a set time, and starvation is a state of involuntary deprivation of food or nutrients.

Fasting is a controlled and intentional process, and when you fast safely, you have enough excess body fat to support the fast. It's important to realize that most of us have enough excess body fat to sustain us for weeks, if not months, of fasting. You're not starving if you have excess body fat; it's as simple as that. As Dr. Now from the TV show *My 600-lb Life* famously said when he was addressing a morbidly obese patient who was scared she was going to starve by skipping a meal, "You have eaten all the food you need for the next four years ahead of time."

Starvation happens when your body has used all its stored body fat and reserves and must therefore start to break down your vital organs and muscles for energy. When you're fasting, if you ever feel the need to break your fast, you can do so; however, if you're starving, you don't have this choice.

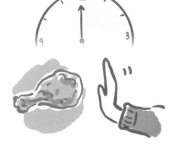

Starvation often results from being put in a vulnerable situation, such as when a person is experiencing poor socioeconomic conditions or neglect and abuse. In these cases, access to food is often beyond the person's control. Starvation usually involves long periods without adequate nutrition, which leads to severe health consequences.

THEY HAVE DIFFERENT PHYSIOLOGICAL EFFECTS

Fasting causes completely different physiological effects than starving. Fasting has many different and well-documented health benefits: It will improve your insulin sensitivity, help you lose excess weight, and improve your brain function. Starvation, on the other hand, can lead to serious consequences for your health, such as malnutrition and organ failure.

The key difference is what happens in your body during fasting versus during starvation. During fasting, your body enters a state of ketosis, where it burns your stored body fat for fuel instead of glucose. As I mentioned earlier, this is a natural process that happens when your body runs out of glucose from food, and it's literally what your body was designed to do. Why else would human beings have evolved to store fat if nature intended us to burn our muscles instead? Think about that for a second. That just doesn't make sense.

In starvation, your body doesn't have enough body fat to burn, so it has to turn to burning your vital organs and muscles.

STARVATION IS A RESULT OF SCARCITY OF FOOD

Another difference between fasting and starving is that when people are starving, they're not necessarily completely starved of food, but it's scarce. They might get a little bit of food once in a while, but sufficient food may never be available. In the case of fasting that's done safely and appropriately, you don't have to worry about food insufficiency. There's always sufficient nutritionally balanced food available for you when you choose to break your fast. Choosing not to eat at all (fasting) is not the same as being able to eat only a very little (starving), because the complete absence of food during fasting activates entirely different processes in your body.

When access to food is scarce but not gone completely, your body lowers its metabolic rate to try to match the limited food intake. However, when you completely restrict food through fasting, it triggers your body to switch to burning stored body fat for fuel, meaning it doesn't have to decrease metabolism.

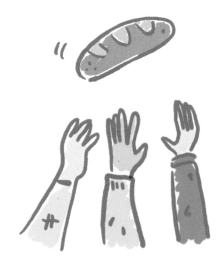

THE MINNESOTA STARVATION EXPERIMENT

The Minnesota Starvation Experiment demonstrated what happens in your body when you're starving. The aim of the experiment was to understand the physical and psychological effects of starvation to help rehabilitate people affected by hunger because of World War II. Thirty-six volunteers were to eat a semi-starvation diet for six months. They ate around 1,500 calories per day, which was roughly half their normal food intake. The participants did not respond well to these conditions, and their health quickly got worse.[1]

Physically, the participants suffered from fatigue, decreases in body temperature, and decreases in muscle mass. Psychologically, they showed signs of anxiety and depression. The participants also became obsessed with food during the experiment—they would talk and dream about it, and they showed abnormal eating behaviors both during the experiment and after it had concluded.[2] The experiment shows that severe caloric restriction, or starvation, can have severely damaging physical and mental consequences.

However, the Minnesota Starvation Experiment doesn't actually illustrate what happens when you're *fasting*. Fasting, when practiced in a controlled and safe way, doesn't involve the severe caloric restriction that the participants were put through in the Minnesota experiment. Fasting involves periods of not eating at all, followed by periods of nourishing your body properly, and that's the key difference here. When you approach fasting in this way, making sure that you refeed carefully and nutritiously, you prevent the serious health consequences associated with starvation.[3]

Humans Evolved to Fast

Humans have often had to adapt to periods when food wasn't readily available. We would often go through so-called fast-and-feast cycles, meaning there would be periods when we had a lot of food available so we ate a lot, and there would be periods when there wasn't any food available, so we didn't eat.

Our hunter-gatherer ancestors, for example, would hunt a big animal and then eat in abundance for a few days: This is what's known as the feast. When that food source was depleted, the hunt for food would begin again, and it might take days or even weeks before they found another animal to eat. This is what's known as the fast. Our ancestors experienced frequent intermittent fasting because they didn't always have a steady supply of food, so their bodies were well adjusted to it. Adapting in this way allowed their bodies to store energy as body fat and use it for fuel when no food was coming in. Your body can also function this way: Think of your body fat as your own super portable lunch box.

Today, however, food is fast, convenient, and available 24/7. Consequently, our bodies have lost this natural access to the fast-and-feast cycle. Instead, we often find ourselves in a constant state of feeding, going from meal to meal and snack to snack, which can lead to several different metabolic disorders and weight gain in the long run. Reintroducing yourself to intermittent fasting allows you to tap in to this evolutionary adaptation. Getting back to those periods of fasting and feasting restores your hormonal balance and promotes a whole host of other health benefits at the same time. So don't let fasting scare you; it's literally what your body was designed to do.

Perhaps the best example for demonstrating that human beings are designed to run on body fat and that we don't die by skipping a few meals is the case of Angus Barbieri.

Barbieri was a Scottish man who fasted for a full 382 days in the 1960s. You read that right. He went 1 year and 17 days completely without food. At 456 pounds, Barbieri was morbidly obese, and he used fasting as a way to get back to a normal body weight.

Research has shown that most people have enough excess body fat to support at least one month of an extended fast; and obese individuals, who have a higher amount of excess body fat, are theoretically able to support a fast of up to six months or longer.[4] Being morbidly obese gave Barbieri's body enough fat reserves to support such a long fast. Barbieri consumed nothing but water, vitamins, and electrolytes throughout his fast, and he received medical supervision to make sure he was safe and didn't suffer from any adverse side effects.[5]

At the end of his fast, Barbieri had gone from 456 pounds to 180 pounds (a 276-pound loss), and he was perfectly healthy throughout the entire process. Barbieri's fast shows how effective fasting can be for weight loss and also highlights something we often forget—human beings are designed to use stored body fat to give us energy when there's no food around.

In 1971, Barbieri's fast was recognized in the *Guinness Book of World Records* as the longest fast ever completed.[6]

Note that although it's true that the human body can manage for long periods without food, a long fast like this one should never be attempted without medical supervision. Extended fasts can be dangerous if not done safely.

The BENEFITS of FASTING

There are many benefits to fasting that go way beyond weight loss. Fasting can have great physical, mental, and emotional benefits too. In this section, I go through some of the most notable benefits of fasting.

It Improves Insulin Sensitivity

One of the main benefits of fasting is that it can improve your insulin sensitivity. In general, insulin sensitivity refers to your body's ability to use insulin effectively to lower blood sugar levels after eating. Having healthy insulin sensitivity is necessary for you to have normal blood sugar values and reduces the risk that you'll develop metabolic disorders.

As I've described previously, eating food, and especially carbohydrates, causes your blood sugar levels to rise. And as a result of more sugar in your blood, your pancreas produces insulin to help your cells use that sugar for immediate energy or as storage in the form of body fat. When you overeat or constantly snack on high-carbohydrate foods, insulin levels stay elevated, which can cause your cells to become insulin resistant.

It's similar to bacteria becoming resistant to antibiotics when you overuse them. After too many bouts of antibiotics, the bacteria that cause you to become sick develop a tolerance, or resistance, and the same level of antibiotics no longer has an effect. The same thing happens with insulin in your body. When you trigger too much insulin to be released too frequently, your body builds up a "tolerance" and needs more and more insulin for your cells to react to it. This level of insulin "burnout" is what we call *insulin resistance*, which is generally the precursor to developing type 2 diabetes.

Fasting breaks the vicious cycle because it drastically reduces your insulin levels. If you can lower your insulin levels frequently enough and for long enough, you'll have improved insulin sensitivity, which can completely reverse your insulin resistance and in turn your risk of developing type 2 diabetes.

It Improves Memory, Brain Function, and Mood

Fasting is not only great for hormonal regulation, but it can also help you improve your brain, including your memory, brain function, and mood.

Research has shown that fasting regularly can help increase brain function as you get older. Intermittent fasting has been shown to improve signs of mild cognitive impairment (MCI), which is a precursor to more severe cases of cognitive decline, such as dementia. One study looked at people over the age of 60 with already established MCI. In the study, the individuals were instructed to try intermittent fasting to see whether it could have an impact on their cognitive function. The study found that those who fasted more often showed a much better cognitive function than those who fasted less or not at all.[7] This suggests that fasting could reverse or slow mild cognitive impairment. These cognitive benefits are likely linked to some biochemical changes caused by fasting, such as raised levels of certain protective enzymes, as well as an increase in ketones, which has been found to protect your brain function and brain health.

Fasting also has a positive effect on your memory because it encourages new brain cells to be produced in the hippocampus, which is a key memory region in the brain. Although most of the existing research has been done on mice, early human studies support that intermittent fasting can improve memory function in humans too.[8]

Studies have also shown that fasting can reduce stress, anxiety, and depression, and it's common to experience increased mental focus and alertness during fasting.[9] This may sound counterintuitive because a lot of people believe that eating food makes you more alert and energetic, but going completely without food, or fasting, can actually increase your concentration and focus.

It Reduces Inflammation

Inflammation is a natural and important part of your body's immune system. It helps your body react to and get rid of injuries and infection, and it usually shows up in the form of redness, heat, swelling, bloating, and pain. While short-term inflammation is important for healing, having chronic inflammation can cause major chronic conditions, such as problems with your cardiovascular system, diabetes, cancer, and neurodegenerative disorders. Chronic inflammation is often caused, or made worse, by lifestyle choices such as a poor diet, lack of exercise, and having chronic stress.

Fasting has been shown to lower inflammation in the body through reducing oxidative stress, which is when there's an imbalance between the number of free radicals and antioxidants in your body, which can be damaging for your cells and tissues. Fasting helps you produce more antioxidants.

Another way fasting helps to reduce inflammation is through autophagy. As I previously mentioned, autophagy is a process where the body gets rid of old and damaged cells—including damaged cells that can be causing inflammation—and produces new ones.

Fasting also reduces inflammation through ketosis. As previously mentioned, ketones are produced through the breakdown of your body fat when you're fasting or eating a low-carbohydrate or ketogenic diet. Ketones have been found to have anti-inflammatory properties, and they can help reduce oxidative stress and inflammation in the body.

One last way fasting can help reduce inflammation in the body is through regulating your gut microbiome—removing bad bacteria and encouraging good bacteria to grow. Having a balanced gut microbiome can help prevent chronic inflammation.

Studies have confirmed the various ways fasting contributes to reduced inflammation. One study found that fasting reduced inflammation and symptoms in patients with rheumatoid arthritis, which is an autoimmune condition characterized by chronic inflammation in the body.[10] Another study looked at how fasting affected people with asthma. The study showed that fasting had a positive effect on reducing oxidative stress as well as inflammatory markers in patients and improved both lung function and asthma symptoms.[11] And finally, two studies found that fasting reduced inflammatory markers and oxidative stress in overweight and obese individuals.[12]

It Improves Gut Health

Another huge benefit of fasting is how it can affect your gut. Fasting has been shown to have a positive effect on both your gut microbiome and your hormonal balance. Having a healthy gut microbiome is important and has many benefits, including improved digestion and nutrient absorption, reduced inflammation, improved immunity, and better mental health.

Your gut contains trillions of bacteria, fungi, viruses, and other microbes. All these microbes are important for taking care of physiological functions and maintaining your gut health. Having a balanced gut microbiome helps with digestion, protects against diseases, helps to break down vitamins appropriately, and helps you have a strong immune system.

Fasting helps you develop a good gut microbiome by promoting the growth of good bacteria in the gut and reducing the growth of bad bacteria. Because fasting provides a rest period for the gut when you're not eating, the gut lining can regenerate and repair itself. This process improves the function of the gut barrier and reduces inflammation.

In fact, research has shown that intermittent fasting can change the makeup and function of your gut microbiome. One study found that changes in the microbiome from fasting can prevent obesity and metabolic syndrome by encouraging the growth of the healthy bacteria that produces short-chain fatty acids.[13] Short-chain fatty acids are important for protecting the lining of the gut and also have anti-inflammatory properties.

It Supercharges Fat Loss While Preserving Muscle Mass

Another benefit to fasting is that it makes you lose body fat while at the same time keeping your muscles safe from breakdown. Preserving your muscles when you're losing weight is important because muscle keeps your metabolism high. This preservation of muscle mass makes fasting different from caloric restriction, which has been found to reduce your muscle mass.[14] Research has also shown that fasting increases fat-burning compared to eating (even a healthy diet), and the longer you fast, the higher the rate of fat-burning becomes.[15]

There are several reasons why fasting helps protect your muscles when you're losing weight. The first one is that it promotes the release of human growth hormone (HGH), which plays an important role in preserving lean muscle mass and promoting fat-burning. When human growth hormone is high, it helps your body burn your stored body fat while at the same time protecting your muscles from being broken down and used as an energy source.

Secondly, fasting protects lean muscle mass because of the production of ketones. Ketones give your body a constant source of energy without food but also have muscle-sparing effects. Ketones help to reduce the breakdown of muscle proteins for gluconeogenesis (where the body produces glucose from noncarbohydrate sources like muscles and body tissue).

Finally, fasting helps to protect muscle mass by improving insulin sensitivity. Improved insulin sensitivity ensures that the nutrients you consume through food are more likely to be used for your muscle cells rather than fat cells, which will make it easier for you to both build and maintain muscle.

The best way to maintain your muscles while losing weight through fasting is to eat a protein-rich diet in your eating window and incorporate resistance training into your exercise routine.

It's Easy to Follow

A huge benefit to fasting that sets it apart from traditional "diets" is that it's super easy to follow. In fact, this was one of the main factors behind my choice to make fasting my way of life. I had never been able to stick to any other diet or lifestyle changes consistently because they made me miserable. I found fasting to be different.

Fasting, at its core, is simple. You choose a period of time (be it a set number of hours or a set number of days) during which you don't eat. That's it. There are no complicated rules to follow and no complicated diets. Just don't eat for certain periods of time, and then make sure you fuel your body with healthy foods when you do eat.

Fasting can easily fit into your busy lifestyle, and you can fast around family and social events if you need to. Never in my life have I been able to lose weight as effortlessly as when I finally cracked the code on fasting. The beauty is that fasting does all the work for you, and you don't even have to step foot in the gym. You can literally be lounging around on the couch all day while watching Netflix, and fasting will be melting your fat off in the background. I'm certainly no gym rat, and I lost all my 40 pounds through fasting without stepping foot in the gym. Easy, healthy, and straightforward—that's why I love it.

Now that you know the basics behind why and how fasting works, it's time to cover the practical aspect of fasting—namely, how to do it. In Chapter 2, I go over the most common fasting schedules so that you know exactly where to begin on your fasting journey.

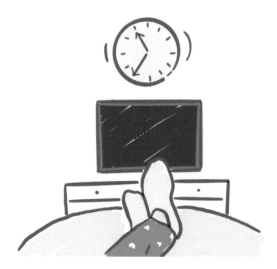

CHAPTER 2
TYPES OF FASTS

Before you get started with fasting, it can be helpful to look at some of the most common fasting schedules to decide which one is the best fit for you.

Many different intermittent and extended fasting schedules exist. They range from sixteen-hour fasts to extended fasting of twenty-four hours or longer. Shorter fasting schedules are great for beginners, whereas longer fasting schedules can provide more benefits but are better suited for more experienced fasters.

In general, the longer you fast, the more weight you'll lose. Shorter fasts also help you lose weight, but your progress will be a little bit slower. That being said, the best fasting schedule is the one you can stick to. It's better to pick a shorter fast and actually complete it than to pick a longer fast and give up.

INTERMITTENT FASTING

Intermittent fasting is probably the most well-known term, and you've most likely heard it thrown around frequently. But what does it mean? Intermittent fasting isn't just one specific schedule. It includes a variety of fasting schedules, including 16:8 (where you fast for sixteen hours and eat for eight), OMAD (where you eat just one meal a day), and alternate-day fasting (or ADF, where you typically eat two meals every thirty-six to forty-two hours).

16:8

16:8 is one of the most popular and well-known intermittent fasting schedules. It involves fasting for sixteen hours each day, followed by an eight-hour eating window. During the fasting window, you have only water, black coffee, and plain tea. (This is true for the fasting windows for all the options.) During the eating window, you eat two meals—usually lunch and dinner or breakfast and lunch.

16:8 is a relatively easy schedule to follow, and it can easily be adapted to fit different lifestyles and preferences. For example, you may have your last meal of the day at 8:00 p.m. and then have your next meal at noon the next day, giving you a sixteen-hour fasting window between 8:00 p.m. and 12:00 p.m.

16:8

	sunday	monday	tuesday	wednesday	thursday	friday	saturday
midnight							
4:00 a.m.	fast	fast	fast	fast	fast	fast	fast
8:00 a.m.							
12:00 p.m.	meal 1	meal 1	meal 1	meal 1	meal 1	meal 1	meal 1
4:00 p.m.							
8:00 p.m.	meal 2	meal 2	meal 2	meal 2	meal 2	meal 2	meal 2
midnight							

Most people can get used to the 16:8 schedule in a short period and lose weight without feeling too hungry. The benefit of the 16:8 schedule is that even though it's easy to follow, you can still see good results. Research has shown that 16:8 can help people lose weight, improve insulin resistance, reduce inflammation, and lower blood pressure while still retaining muscle mass.[1]

Fasting for sixteen hours can seem daunting at first, but keep in mind that you spend much of that time sleeping. For example, if you finish dinner at 8:00 p.m. and don't eat again until noon the next day, you've already completed more than half of your fast by the time you wake up in the morning. This makes 16:8 a lot more manageable than it looks at first glance.

However, if you want to get the benefits of autophagy, 16:8 might not be for you because autophagy begins at around twenty-four hours of fasting. Another possible disadvantage of the 16:8 schedule is that you may not lose weight as quickly as following a longer fasting schedule.

Despite the possible disadvantages, 16:8 is a great option if you're new to fasting or prefer eating out with friends and family on a regular basis. Once you've gotten used to 16:8, you can move on to the 18:6 schedule and build up your fasting hours from there. With 18:6, you extend your fasting window and eat your two meals within a six-hour window instead of an eight-hour window.

OMAD

OMAD is short for "one meal a day," and, as the name suggests, you eat just one meal every twenty-four hours when you're on this schedule. Once your meal is finished, you restart your fasting timer and start another twenty-four-hour fast. Most people choose to have dinner as their one meal because it usually makes it easier to handle family life and social events, but you can have your meal at any time convenient for you. For example, if you have your OMAD at 6:00 p.m., you would fast until 6:00 p.m. the next day.

OMAD is a more advanced form of intermittent fasting than 16:8, but most people still get used to it pretty easily after a few days, and they begin to feel less hungry throughout the day.

One of the main advantages of OMAD is its simplicity. Many people find it easier to stick to a simple eating schedule rather than thinking about several meal preparations and food selections throughout the day. With OMAD, there's no need to count calories or constantly plan your meals for the day. You eat just once, and that's it.

Some people suggest that to do OMAD correctly, you need to eat all your daily calories during your one meal. However, if fasting has taught me anything, it's to listen to my body. Make sure you pick a healthy, nutrient-dense meal for OMAD and eat until you're satisfied, but never force yourself to eat. One of the main benefits of intermittent fasting is that it can teach you to tune in to your true hunger and fullness cues.

OMAD is great for weight loss. The long fasting window puts your body into ketosis, where it breaks down your stored body fat into ketones for fuel. On top of that, because you have just one meal each day, you keep your insulin levels low for the majority of the day, which means OMAD can improve insulin sensitivity and regulate blood sugar levels, which are important for preventing or managing conditions like diabetes.

Other than weight loss and metabolic benefits, OMAD can also improve your mental clarity and focus. When your body is no longer digesting food throughout the day, it has more energy for other things. Many people who use OMAD every day feel more alert and productive during their fasting periods.

A potential disadvantage of OMAD is that it may be difficult for some people to go a whole day without eating. If you struggle with OMAD, try easing into it by progressively extending your fast until you can spend most of the day without eating. The more you fast, the easier it will become.

OMAD

	sunday	monday	tuesday	wednesday	thursday	friday	saturday
midnight							
4:00 a.m.	fast	fast	fast	fast	fast	fast	fast
8:00 a.m.							
12:00 p.m.							
4:00 p.m.							
	meal	meal	meal	meal	meal	meal	meal
8:00 p.m.							
midnight	fast	fast	fast	fast	fast	fast	fast

ADF

As the name suggests, alternate-day fasting (ADF) involves fasting every other day. On ADF, you do a thirty-six- to forty-two-hour fast from dinner one day until breakfast or lunch thirty-six or so hours later (not eating at all on the day after your dinner). For example, if you have dinner at 8:00 p.m. you fast all throughout the following day. The day after that, you eat lunch at 12:00 p.m. and dinner at 8:00 p.m., and then repeat the pattern.

Because of the length of the fasting period, ADF is one of the most effective forms of intermittent fasting when it comes to both health and weight loss. This schedule helps you regulate your blood sugar levels, lower your blood pressure, and more.[2] Studies have also shown that ADF is great for increasing autophagy, and even increasing your lifespan.[3]

However, for some people, ADF can be a bit more challenging than the other forms of intermittent fasting because of the longer fasting hours. But research has shown that ADF can be a hugely effective strategy for losing weight, reducing body fat, and improving cholesterol levels.[4]

Despite the potentially challenging schedule, the cyclical nature of ADF helps some people stick to it more effectively than traditional low-calorie diet plans. On traditional low-calorie diets, you consistently eat less than you need or want. But with ADF (and intermittent fasting in general), you don't eat at all for a period of time, but eat until satisfaction when you do eat.

ADF	sunday	monday	tuesday	wednesday	thursday	friday	saturday
midnight							
4:00 a.m.	fast		fast		fast		fast
8:00 a.m.							
12:00 p.m.	meal 1	fast	meal 1	fast	meal 1	fast	meal 1
4:00 p.m.							
8:00 p.m.	meal 2		meal 2		meal 2		meal 2
midnight							

ROLLING 48s

Rolling 48s is a more challenging fasting plan than the intermittent fasting options I've already described in this chapter. When you're on a rolling 48 schedule, you eat just one meal every forty-eight hours.

Because the fasting period is longer, you need to have more discipline and dedication, but you may realize more benefits in terms of weight loss and metabolic shifts.

Rather than limiting yourself to a set eating window every day, you enjoy one meal every forty-eight hours. Most people have their one meal at the same time every other day, usually at dinner, but you can adjust your schedule if you need to. This means you can have your meal at a time that's convenient for you, making it easy to incorporate into your daily routine. For example, you'd eat dinner on Monday night at 7:00 p.m., and then you wouldn't eat again until dinner at 7:00 p.m. on Wednesday night.

Rolling 48s has many benefits for your body because of the longer fasting window and the metabolic adaptations it causes. One advantage is that it puts your body through autophagy, which is great for your cellular health.

When you're doing rolling 48s, you're also maximizing the benefits of ketosis because you give your body plenty of time to fully enter ketosis and experience all its fat-burning benefits.

Longer fasts like this can also improve your insulin sensitivity and blood sugar levels. Forty-eight-hour fasts have been shown to improve insulin sensitivity significantly in those with insulin resistance.[5] Improving insulin sensitivity helps manage blood sugar levels, which is important for those who either have or are at risk of developing type 2 diabetes; keeping blood sugar levels low reduces the need for medication.

Aside from the physical benefits, forty-eight-hour fasts have been linked to improved mood, mental clarity, and cognitive function.[6]

When you're on a rolling 48s schedule, make sure you drink plenty of water and eat a high-quality, nutrient-dense meal when you break your fast.

ROLLING 48s

1ST WEEK

	sunday	monday	tuesday	wednesday	thursday	friday	saturday
midnight							
4:00 a.m.	fast		fast		fast		fast
8:00 a.m.							
12:00 p.m.		fast		fast		fast	
4:00 p.m.							
8:00 p.m.	meal		meal		meal		meal
midnight	fast		fast		fast		fast

2ND WEEK

	sunday	monday	tuesday	wednesday	thursday	friday	saturday
midnight							
4:00 a.m.		fast		fast		fast	
8:00 a.m.							
12:00 p.m.	fast		fast		fast		fast
4:00 p.m.							
8:00 p.m.		meal		meal		meal	
midnight		fast		fast		fast	

5:2

The 5:2 fasting schedule is an advanced kind of intermittent fasting that goes further than the traditional intermittent fasting schedules. It's perfect if you want to challenge yourself and see rapid weight loss and greater health benefits.

The 5:2 schedule involves fasting for five full days, followed by a two-day eating window. This is not the same as the more conventional 5:2 method, which involves eating fewer calories (typically no more than 500 calories) on two nonconsecutive days and eating normally for the five remaining days of the week. On the 5:2 fasting schedule, you would usually fast from Monday to Friday and then eat either one or two meals per day on Saturday and Sunday.

Because of its extended fasting phase, the 5:2 fasting schedule has the potential to trigger a wide range of physiological benefits. Extended fasting maximizes autophagy and insulin sensitivity, which is an important factor in lowering your risk of weight gain and developing type 2 diabetes.[7]

Extended fasting triggers the breakdown of stored body fat for energy,[8] so one of the most appealing aspects of the 5:2 fasting schedule is that it's super effective in terms of weight loss and fat-burning.

Although the potential benefits of 5:2 fasting are great, you should always be careful when you're doing any type of extended fasting and consult a medical professional before attempting it.

5:2

	sunday	monday	tuesday	wednesday	thursday	friday	saturday
midnight							
4:00 a.m.							
8:00 a.m.						fast	fast
12:00 p.m.	fast	fast	fast	fast	fast		
4:00 p.m.							
8:00 p.m.						meal	meal
midnight						fast	fast

EXTENDED FASTING

Once you move beyond the 5:2 schedule, you're really getting into the most challenging form of fasting. Extended fasting refers to fasting for extended periods of time, usually anything from forty-eight hours to several days or even weeks at a time.

This type of fasting requires more discipline and planning, and in some cases, you shouldn't do it without medical supervision. When done correctly, it can provide many health benefits, including weight loss, improved brain function, decreased inflammation, increased cellular repair, increased longevity, increased insulin sensitivity, and improved health.[9]

One of the biggest pros of extended fasting is that you'll lose a significant amount of weight. In fact, extended fasting is the most effective weight-loss schedule because you spend a long time in ketosis, or fat-burning mode. According to one study in 2023, fasting for five days resulted in a 4 to 6 percent weight loss; fasting for seven to ten days resulted in a 2 to 10 percent weight loss; and fasting for 15 to 20 days resulted in a 7 to 10 percent weight loss.[10] As a general rule, the longer you fast, the more fat you'll burn, and the more weight you'll lose.[11]

Another benefit of extended fasting is that it maximizes autophagy, which you may recall is the process by which the body gets rid of damaged cells and waste. By not eating for an extended period, autophagy is not only activated but sustained. Several studies have shown that autophagy is important for your general health and lifespan. For example, autophagy plays an important role in preventing age-related illnesses such as Alzheimer's disease, Parkinson's disease, and cancer.[12] People who practice extended fasting tend to have lower levels of inflammation, which means extended fasting makes you healthier overall.[13] Extended fasting also increases the production of human growth hormone (HGH), which helps you burn more fat while at the same time protecting your muscles.[14]

Although the benefits of extended fasting can be great, you should approach any long fasts carefully. Always make sure that you eat balanced, low-carb, and nutrient-dense meals in preparation for an extended fast. Your pre-fast meals should include all necessary vitamins, minerals, and macronutrients to keep you healthy during the fast. You can sometimes experience some uncomfortable side effects, such as headaches or nausea, when you're on an extended fast, but those symptoms are usually just a sign that you're low in electrolytes, so as long as you're mindful of getting enough electrolytes, you should be fine. I outline the electrolyte requirements for fasting later in the book.

Note: Extended fasting is not for everyone, especially if you have underlying health conditions or you're new to fasting. Always ask your doctor if fasting is right for you.

FASTING and PERIODS

You may feel hungrier at certain points of your cycle or struggle with cravings or low moods. Because of this, some experts suggest that you should adjust your fasting schedule according to the phase of your menstrual cycle. But is this really the case?

The first half of the menstrual cycle is the follicular phase when estrogen increases. It usually starts at the beginning of menstruation and lasts until ovulation. During this phase, some individuals experience increased energy levels and reduced cravings, which can make fasting easier to tolerate.

The second half of the menstrual cycle is the luteal phase, when progesterone levels increase. This phase starts right after ovulation and ends when the next menstrual cycle begins. In the luteal phase, you might experience increased appetite, water retention, and mood swings. These factors may make fasting more challenging.

Because of these hormonal changes, some experts advise adjusting your fasting schedules based on where in the menstrual cycle you are. They suggest that in the follicular phase, when appetite is decreased and mood is more stable, you should increase your fasting hours. In the luteal phase, when cravings and water retention are higher, they say you should fast less or not at all.

I think these recommendations overcomplicate what is really a very simple process. I don't adjust my fasting schedule based on my period or cycle, and I have never advised any of my clients to do so either. The main reason fasting is so appealing to me is because of how simple it is. You don't need to track calories or macros or stick to any complicated meal plans. You fast, and then you eat. So having to stick to complicated rules, schedules, and timing based on your menstrual cycle defeats this whole purpose.

Furthermore, I know our ancient ancestors didn't use apps to track their cycles, and they didn't limit hunting for animals to their luteal phase. They ate when they had food and didn't eat when they didn't. There was a balance between fasting and feasting that kept human beings healthy, without tracking any macros, calories, or cycles. Human beings were made to fast—that's why we have the functionality to store and use body fat. I have always fasted through my periods, and it has worked great for me. So my recommendation is to pick a fasting schedule that you're comfortable with and stick with it. Fasting is simple, healthy, and highly effective for fat loss. There's no need to overcomplicate it.

Chapter 3 dives into the history of our modern eating habits. In it, I explain why so many people struggle with weight gain and why eating a low-fat diet is the worst thing you can do if you want to create sustainable weight loss.

CHAPTER 3
WHY MODERN LIFE HAS LED TO AN OBESITY EPIDEMIC

You might be surprised to find out that before our modern-day obsession with calorie counting, people had a more intuitive understanding of the relationship between weight gain and food—specifically the role carbohydrates play in weight gain. Over time, however, it seems that this intuitive knowledge has slowly disappeared. In this chapter, I talk about how we got to where we are today and discuss how modern life has contributed to an obesity epidemic.

HOW IT USED to BE

One of the earliest works on food and diet, the book *The Physiology of Taste: Or Meditations on Transcendental Gastronomy with Recipes* written by Jean Anthelme Brillat-Savarin and published in 1825, talks about the effect that different types of food have on the body.

This book was the foundation for starting to understand how diet affects our health and weight. Brillat-Savarin found that people who ate bread and other products made with flour were more likely to gain weight, whereas people who focused on eating proteins and fats did not.[1]

Later in the nineteenth century, William Banting, an English undertaker, also looked at the relationship between eating a high-carbohydrate diet and weight gain. Banting had struggled with obesity for most of his life. He'd tried several different diets and weight-loss methods, but nothing had worked for him. After many failed attempts at getting his weight under control, Banting approached a doctor who, contrary to popular practice at the time, put him on a diet low in carbohydrates and high in protein and fats.

Banting lost a significant amount of weight, going from 202 pounds to 156 pounds. In 1863, he published a pamphlet: "Letter on Corpulence, Addressed to the Public."[2] In this pamphlet, Banting talked about the diet he followed to lose weight, which mainly consisted of meat, fish, and vegetables and completely cut out sugar, starches, beer, and dairy. His pamphlet was ground-breaking because it shifted people's focus from simply eating less to lose weight to changing the types of foods they ate. Banting's pamphlet and his dramatic weight loss had a huge influence on dietary practices at the time. His pamphlet became a bestseller, was translated into many different languages, and influenced dietary recommendations and practices all over the world. It has been described as the first diet book ever published, and his approach laid the groundwork for many of the low-carbohydrate diets we see today, highlighting how processed carbs and sugar cause us to gain weight. In fact, Banting became so strongly associated with weight loss that the word *banting* is still used in several languages, including my native Sweden, to refer to "going on a diet."

Unfortunately, somewhere along the way, Banting's wisdom seems to have been forgotten. In modern society, and for several decades past, the advice on weight loss has been to "eat less and move more" or simply to eat less fat. What's important to understand is that when you remove fat from a product, it becomes a lot less tasty. To offset the reduced flavor, food manufacturers add more sugar and carbs to low-fat products so that people will want to eat them. And if Banting's pamphlet offers any clues, it's that low-fat and high-carbohydrate "diet" products only lead to weight gain in the long run.

What's promising is that the principles suggested by Brillat-Savarin and Banting are now supported by scientific research. Several studies have shown that low-carb diets can make you lose weight and improve your metabolic health. One study found that people who were put on a low-carbohydrate diet lost more weight and experienced better cardiovascular health than people who were put on a low-fat diet.[3]

Over the roughly 100 years following Brillat-Savarin and Banting's teachings, up until the 1950s, low-carb, high-protein, high-fat diets were widely accepted as the best way to lose weight. If you wanted to lose weight, you would simply stop eating so much sugar and bread. Just ask your grandparents.

In the 1940s and '50s, the typical American diet had a lot of hearty breakfast options, including eggs, bacon, and other high-protein and high-fat foods. The general idea was that these types of meals were able to give you sustained energy throughout the day, and they were common staples in households across the country. Back then, people inherently understood that high-carb foods such as bread, pastries, and cookies caused you to gain weight, and there was a more commonsense approach to eating that focused on the quality of food rather than counting calories. That's something that we've completely lost today.

CHANGING DIETS and the LOW-FAT MOVEMENT

Then attitudes about fatty foods changed in the 1950s. The reason for this shift was a dramatic increase in heart disease across the country, and people were desperate to find the culprit.

During the next couple of decades, several very influential but also controversial studies painted dietary fat as the main cause of heart disease. One of the most famous studies that linked saturated fat intake to cardiovascular disease was Ancel Keys's Seven Countries Study from 1970, which spanned several decades starting in the late '50s. This (flawed) study looked at fat and carbohydrate intake across various countries around the world and compared it to the number of deaths from heart disease in those same countries. However, Keys cherry-picked his data and included only the countries that supported his hypothesis: the United States, Japan, Yugoslavia, the Netherlands, Finland, Greece, and Italy. His hypothesis was true in those countries. But he conveniently left out fifteen other countries—including the Nordic countries of Sweden, Denmark, and Norway—where people ate quite a lot of fat but heart disease deaths were relatively few. He also omitted Chile, which had a lot of cardiovascular deaths despite having a relatively low consumption of fat. On these shaky grounds, fat was painted as the villain that needed to be eradicated by any means necessary.

The American Heart Association (AHA) also promoted the low-fat diet. In the 1960s and '70s, the AHA provided guidelines that pointed to dietary fat as the main cause of heart disease. These guidelines suggested that reducing dietary fat intake would lower the level of harmful cholesterol and therefore reduce the risk of heart disease. Yet subsequent research has questioned these findings, and it has been suggested that the focus on reducing dietary fat was actually seriously wrong.

One of the reasons why these conclusions are flawed is that they disregard the impact of life expectancy. In 1900, the life expectancy (for men) was 48 years. In 1950, it was 67 years; by 1970, it was more than 70 years.[4] In the early 1900s, people were dying of all kinds of diseases, such as tuberculosis, pneumonia, diarrhea, and enteritis. But with the development of modern medicine, vaccines, and better hygiene, life expectancy started to dramatically increase. The fact is, the older a person gets, the more likely they are to experience a heart attack. And if people weren't dying at earlier ages from infections or vaccine-treatable diseases, more and more people were living long enough to die from heart attacks. The average age for a heart attack (for men) is 65 years.[5] The risk of a heart attack is much lower for someone who is 50 years old than for someone who is 65 years old, so it's only natural that an overall increase in life expectancy resulted in an overall increase in heart attacks, regardless of diet. So dietary fat was given a bad rap for no reason.

But with Keys's study linking fat to heart disease, together with the guidelines from the AMA, there was a huge shift in eating patterns among the American public. People went from eating the standard high-fat, high-protein diet to a low-fat, high-carbohydrate diet. In 1977, the low-fat diet movement exploded when the United States Senate Select Committee on Nutrition and Human Needs officially adopted the advice of Ancel Keys and released the Dietary Goals for the United States. The new guidelines suggested that people were to reduce the calories from fat to 30 percent of total calories consumed and increase the calories from carbs to 55 to 60 percent of total calories consumed.[6] The publication of these guidelines was the final nail in the coffin for the traditional dietary advice that focused on the risks of eating refined carbohydrates. But it didn't stop there. As low-fat diets became more popular, snacking and eating multiple meals a day also gained popularity.

Yet, even with this new, supposedly healthier dietary advice, the general population continued to get heavier and heavier. The rate of obesity in 1960 was just 10 percent; by 2018, it had increased to 42 percent.[7]

So the widespread adoption of these low-fat diets and frequent meals and snacks had severe negative consequences for the health of the population. We now know that staying in a constant state of eating causes chronically high insulin levels, making it very difficult for the body to access and burn stored body fat.[8] As I've previously mentioned, when you remove fat from a food—yogurt, for example—you have to add more sugar and other refined carbohydrates to make the food taste even remotely good. This is because fat has flavor, so when you remove the fat, you remove the flavor. Millions of Americans were now obsessed with low-fat and no-fat products, which have been proven to increase obesity, type 2 diabetes, and metabolic syndrome.[9]

In the wake of the new low-fat dietary guidelines, cardiovascular disease and diabetes rates not only didn't decrease, but they kept increasing, suggesting that perhaps the low-fat, high-carbohydrate dietary advice was more than a little flawed. A study published in the

Journal of the American Medical Association supports this suggestion, finding that the dietary changes over the past several decades have not improved cardiovascular health, and obesity and diabetes rates have both continued to skyrocket.[10]

The reason we run into so much trouble is because these guidelines were based on limited and sometimes inconclusive data and conflicting evidence. In the 1970s, John Yudkin, a well-known British nutritionist, was one of the only people to challenge the theory that a low-fat diet is good for your health. He wrote the book *Pure, White and Deadly* in 1972, where he proposed that it was sugar, and not fat, that was responsible for the increasing rates of obesity and heart disease.[11] Unfortunately, his warnings about carbs and sugar were largely ignored at the time.

WHERE WE are TODAY

Even though there's overwhelming evidence against it, the focus on low-fat diets still hasn't gone away. Public health advice and government dietary guidelines still emphasize the importance of low-fat products while downplaying or completely ignoring the harmful effects high levels of processed carbs can have on your body.

Not only has the focus on low-fat diets not solved the obesity epidemic, but it has actually made it worse over time.

Compounding the problem is our frequency of eating, which has increased significantly. It's not uncommon to hear fitness experts and dietitians recommend eating six small meals a day to keep your metabolism high and blood sugar level stable. And snacking is significantly more common now than it was in the 1970s.[12] In fact, more than 90 percent of Americans now eat one to three snacks per day.[13] Snacking is becoming an addiction. Forty-four percent of adults show symptoms of addiction to processed foods, including intense cravings and withdrawals if they don't have access to these foods.[14]

At the same time that these misguided dietary recommendations continue to reign supreme, there's been a shift in society toward normalizing obesity. Although the body positivity movement has done a lot of great work to promote self-love and reduce discrimination against people with bigger bodies, it's also important to be aware of and acknowledge the risks that come with obesity.

Being overweight or obese is not just an aesthetic personal preference. Carrying too much weight on your body is a significant risk factor for developing chronic diseases, such as heart disease, type 2 diabetes, depression, and even some forms of cancer.[15] Celebrating or normalizing obesity without acknowledging what it means for health could lead people into a false sense of security about their weight and stop them from trying to live healthier lives.

And the body positivity movement may also have the unintended consequence of making people more overweight. Some research has shown that spending time with overweight people can increase a person's likelihood of becoming overweight. If your friend becomes overweight, you're 57 percent more likely to become overweight yourself as a result. If your sibling becomes overweight, your risk of becoming overweight increases by 40 percent. If your spouse becomes overweight, your risk of becoming overweight increases by 37 percent.[16]

Another study found that simply looking at a picture of an overweight person can cause you to consume more calories. Participants in this study were presented with a scenario: "Your overweight friend sends you pictures from her vacation. After viewing her pictures, someone in the office walks by offering you a plate of cookies. Will you eat more or fewer cookies after viewing your friend's pictures?" Most people believed they would be inspired to eat fewer cookies after seeing their overweight friend, but the opposite was actually true. After viewing the pictures, participants actually ate more cookies.[17] The idea is that if heavier bodies are seen and celebrated more in the media and society, the consequence will be that more people will gain weight, which will keep moving the goal post of what is seen as a "healthy" or "normal" weight. Seeing more overweight people around you may lead to a false sense of security when it comes to your own weight and might cause you to see yourself and your unhealthy food behaviors as less problematic, which can perpetuate the weight-gain cycle even more.

Despite the overwhelming evidence showing how detrimental high-carb diets and obesity can be when it comes to health, many people are completely unaware of how different foods affect their hormones, gut health, and well-being. This lack of awareness leads people to continue the cycle of bad eating habits and weight struggles.

Luckily, current dietary guidelines have started to take a more balanced approach, emphasizing that eating more unprocessed whole foods and fewer processed carbohydrates and sugars is an important part of a healthy diet. There is also a renewed interest in low-carbohydrate and ketogenic diets as a way to lose weight and stay healthy.

The way you're living today is keeping you overweight and unhealthy. If you want to achieve sustainable weight loss, you have to know how your diet and behaviors affect your body. This involves understanding how different foods affect your hormone levels— especially the hormones responsible for fat storage, hunger, and fullness—as well as understanding how different types of foods affect your gut microbiome. Having this knowledge will ensure that you'll never need to struggle with your weight again.

One of the biggest keys to sustainable weight loss is understanding why the traditional calories in, calories out model doesn't work, and that's what I'll cover in the next chapter.

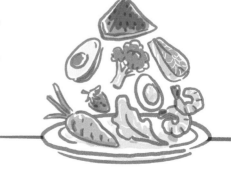

CHAPTER 4
FASTING ISN'T ABOUT CALORIES

One of the key messages I want you to take away from this book is that *fasting is not about calories,* despite what you may have heard before.

When people say that the only reason fasting works is because it reduces the number of calories you eat, they're completely wrong. Fasting creates very different physiological responses in your body compared to simple caloric restriction, and it's important to know about these differences if you want to lose weight effectively.

Diets that focus on caloric restriction tell you to cut down on the number of calories you eat every day. There are many different recommendations; some tell you to cut 500 to 700 calories a day, whereas others recommend that you eat no more than 1,200 calories a day. Even more extreme recommendations tell you to consume no more than 850 calories a day.

When you're on a calorie-restricted diet, you spread your calories evenly throughout the day, usually through eating several small meals. The main focus of caloric restriction is a combination of portion control and keeping up constant but lower levels of food intake.

On the other hand, fasting involves periods of not eating at all followed by periods of eating normally. This type of intermittent fasting can be done daily for short periods of time, such as sixteen hours of fasting with an eight-hour eating window, or longer periods of twenty-four hours or more. With caloric restriction, you eat smaller amounts of food constantly; with fasting, you pair intervals where you don't put any food at all into your system with intervals where you don't restrict.

Your body responds to each of these approaches in different ways. In this chapter, I explain those differences.

COMPARING the BODY'S RESPONSES to CALORIC RESTRICTION and FASTING

Plain and simple, calorie-restricted diets are unsuccessful in the long run, and research has confirmed this. The success rate for standard low-calorie diets is incredibly poor.

A year after losing weight on a low-calorie diet, 95 percent of people regain the weight they lost. And five years later, more than 50 percent will weigh more than they did before they started.[1]

Most of us know this to be true from personal experience. But why does it happen?

When you drastically lower the number of calories you eat, your body responds by reducing your metabolic rate to save energy. This effect, known as metabolic slowdown, makes it more and more difficult for you to lose weight even when you keep lowering your calories. Furthermore, caloric restriction has been shown to lead to increased hunger, which makes it more difficult to maintain a calorie-restricted diet over time.[2]

Fasting creates different physiological responses compared to caloric restriction, and I've broken them down for you in the following sections.

Hormonal Changes

Some significant hormonal changes happen when you fast:

- **Insulin:** Fasting reduces insulin levels, which helps prevent insulin resistance and enables your body to access and burn stored body fat.[3]

- **Noradrenaline:** Fasting increases the level of noradrenaline in your body, which helps your metabolism stay high.[4]

- **Human growth hormone:** Fasting increases the level of human growth hormone in your body, which helps protect your lean muscle mass and increase fat-burning.[5]

- **Ghrelin:** Whereas caloric restriction makes you feel hungrier by increasing the hunger hormone ghrelin, studies have shown that fasting lowers ghrelin over time, decreasing your appetite and making it easier to lose weight.[6]

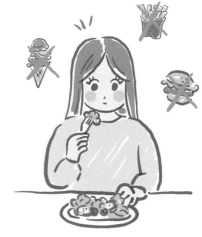

Metabolic Rate

Unlike caloric restriction, fasting doesn't reduce your basal metabolic rate (BMR). In fact, it can increase it, which means your energy levels stay up and you can keep doing your daily activities during fasting.[7]

The reason you often regain weight after you've lost it through caloric restriction is because your metabolism has slowed (and your appetite has increased), but this doesn't happen with fasting. Instead, fasting helps you maintain your metabolism; at the same time, it makes you less hungry and helps you burn more fat.[8] (Read more about this in the next section.)

Fuel Utilization

Fasting causes a switch in how you use energy. At the beginning of your fast, your body uses your liver's glycogen stores for fuel. After these glycogen stores have been depleted, your body starts burning your stored body fat for fuel, which makes you lose weight without affecting your muscle mass.[9]

WHY the "EAT LESS, MOVE MORE" MODEL of WEIGHT LOSS HAS YOU FOOLED

As I mentioned earlier in the "Metabolic Rate" section, caloric restriction leads to weight gain in the long run. In fact, a scientific review done in 2016 showed that fasting helps people lose weight more effectively than low-calorie diets.[10] The traditional advice of "eat less and work out more" is actually more likely to cause short-term weight loss *now* but long-term weight gain *later*. Why does caloric restriction not lead to sustainable weight loss? There are a few different reasons, which I unpack in this section.

Metabolic Slowdown

When you significantly reduce calories, your body slows its metabolism to save energy for survival. This means that as time goes on, your body burns fewer calories at rest. To continue to lose weight, you have to eat less and less food over time, which is not a situation that can be maintained over a long period. When you start eating regularly again, you have a decreased metabolism, and you will regain all the weight you lost and potentially more.[11]

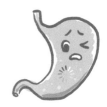

Hormonal Imbalances

Diets with very low calories may affect normal hormonal balances such as ghrelin and leptin, which are responsible for controlling your hunger and fullness cues. Ghrelin increases when you're eating very few calories, making you feel more hungry. Leptin decreases, which makes you feel less satisfied after meals. This disastrous combination makes sustainable weight loss through caloric restriction very difficult.[12]

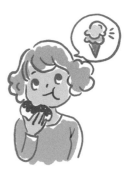

Muscle Loss

Low-calorie diets can result in muscle loss, particularly if you're not eating enough protein. Because muscle is a metabolically active tissue, having less muscle mass makes your resting metabolic rate (the number of calories you burn at rest) lower.[13] When you eventually return to your usual way of eating, you'll burn fewer calories because you have less muscle mass; therefore, you gain more weight.

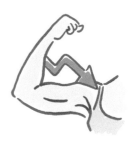

Increased Stress

Overexercising and severe caloric restriction can cause you to feel more stressed, leading to increased production of the stress hormone cortisol. Short-term increases of cortisol are natural and usually nothing to be concerned about, but having long-term elevated cortisol levels can cause you to gain weight. Elevated cortisol levels have been found to increase appetite.[14] Also, they can cause you to gain fat, especially in the stomach area.[15]

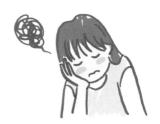

Rebound Overeating

When you severely restrict calories, you may eventually find yourself experiencing binge-eating episodes, which will erase any caloric deficit you achieved on the diet. This restrict-and-binge cycle often leads to weight gain over time.

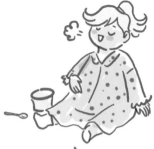

Psychological Toll

The cycle of dieting and weight gain can be demoralizing, and it may lead you to have a negative relationship to food and body image. The negativity can make you less likely to stick to healthy lifestyle choices and increase the likelihood that you'll gain weight.

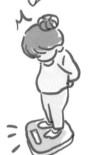

Working Out Won't Make You Lose Weight

Most people think that if you want to lose weight, you have to go to the gym. That's why gym memberships soar in January when everybody wants to get rid of their holiday weight. Although working out is great for a lot of things, like improving your mental health, physical health, and strength, it won't necessarily make you lose weight.

One reason working out doesn't affect weight as much as you might think is that it burns fewer calories than you expect. A thirty-minute gym session burns between 140 and 280 calories (depending on the type of workout you're doing).[16] If you put this into perspective, there are around 300 calories in an apple topped with one tablespoon of peanut butter (or in one Snickers bar). Research shows that moderately exercising for thirty minutes a day, five days a week (which is generally the amount of exercise recommended to maintain good health in adults) doesn't actually produce any meaningful weight loss at all.[17] So instead of killing it for an hour at the gym, you're better off just skipping that extra snack.

In case you still don't believe me, let's look at the numbers. One pound of body fat is around 3,500 calories. If you were to lose weight by working out alone, you would need to burn an extra 500 calories day just to lose a measly one pound per week. Burning those extra calories takes a lot of time and energy. It's easier to cut down on foods or skip a couple of extra snacks rather than trying to burn the same amount of calories through exercise. Not eating a 500-calorie dessert is much easier and more practical than running for an hour every day.

Research confirms that trying to lose weight through exercise alone is highly inefficient, and the best results are achieved by combining diet with exercise.[18] It really is true what they say: *You can't outrun a bad diet.*

Working out can also work against you because it can make you feel hungrier.[19] If you've ever done an intense workout, you might have noticed that you're hungrier afterward. This is because working out can increase your appetite. Therefore, you're likely to eat more calories after working out than if you don't work out at all. Your increased post-workout appetite will probably cancel out the calories you burned during your workout, so at the end of the day, you're running a zero-sum game. The tendency to overestimate the amount of calories you burn through exercise can also be a problem. You might feel like you can "treat yourself" by overeating after a tough gym session, which again will probably cancel out whatever you burned during your workout.

As I mentioned previously, working out can also increase your cortisol levels (your stress hormones), and having constantly high levels of cortisol in your body can make weight loss more difficult. It may even cause you to gain more weight, especially around your stomach.

I'm not making these points to say that you *shouldn't* exercise, of course! Exercise is great, *if it makes you feel good.* Pick an activity you enjoy, don't go too hard, and most important, don't use exercise as an excuse to overeat.

CASE STUDY: *BIGGEST LOSER* CONTESTANTS

One of the best examples of how catastrophic and destructive the "eat less and move more" model can be is the American TV show *The Biggest Loser*. On *The Biggest Loser*, overweight people compete against each other to see who can lose the most weight in a short time. The contestants achieve mind-blowing weight loss through a combination of extreme caloric restriction and intense exercise.

It might surprise you that despite losing massive amounts of weight and transforming their bodies completely, the majority of the contestants from *The Biggest Loser* regain all the weight afterward. But why does this happen?

The basic premise of the show involves putting the participants on a 1,200- to 1,500-calorie diet plan, which is approximately 70 percent less than what their bodies need for energy. This extreme caloric restriction is combined with intense exercise for somewhere between five and eight hours a day.[20] In a six-month period, the participants lose an average of 127 pounds.[21] This has to be proof of the effectiveness of the "eat less, move more" strategy, right? It does work—at least in the short term. Extreme caloric restriction and intense exercise does lead to extreme weight loss in these participants; there's no denying that. Unfortunately, the long-term reality is a very different story.

One of the biggest issues that the participants of *The Biggest Loser* face is metabolic slowdown. Because they're severely restricting their calories and overexercising, their bodies compensate by reducing their resting metabolic rate (RMR), which is the number of calories burned while at rest.[22] For example, when studying the contestants from the show's second season, researchers found that participants had an average decrease in their RMR of 789 calories per day over the course of the show.[23] This means these participants burn 789 fewer calories every day, despite continuing with their diet and exercise routines.

When these participants returned home after the show, their weight loss eventually stalled, and they regained weight gradually because their metabolisms had slowed way down. Despite continuing to follow their low-calorie diet and exercise regimes, their bodies needed fewer and fewer calories because of their reduced RMR, and eventually, cutting calories lower and lower simply becomes unsustainable. The only result is weight gain. One of the contestants from season two of the show, Suzanne Mendonca, was famously quoted as saying that the reason there's never a reunion show for *The Biggest Loser* is that "we're all fat again."[24] Ouch.

Six years after competing on *The Biggest Loser,* most of the participants had regained all the weight they'd lost.[25] Even years later, the participants' metabolisms hadn't fully recovered; their BMR was still 500 calories a day lower than was expected for their body size. This means that even after regaining all of their weight, many of the participants needed to consume significantly fewer calories just to maintain their bigger bodies. Season eight winner Danny Cahill regained most of his weight and now says he has to eat 800 calories less than a man his size typically eats just so he can maintain that high weight.[26] These findings are similar to what Ancel Keys found in the Minnesota Starvation Experiment in the 1950s. As you may remember, the participants in the study saw a 30 percent reduction in their BMR as a response to severe caloric restriction.[27]

And it's not just one or two participants sharing this experience. Many of the former contestants of *The Biggest Loser* have gone on record stating that the show harmed their metabolism and general well-being. For example, Kai Hibbard, who was a contestant on the show's third season, talked about how the show severely damaged her metabolism and how she regained a lot of the weight after the show ended, leading to struggles with her weight as well as her physical and mental health.[28] The first-ever winner of *The Biggest Loser*, Ryan Benson, regained all his weight and, even worse, experienced kidney failure as a result of participating in the show.[29]

The experience of *The Biggest Loser* contestants powerfully highlights why caloric restriction and overexercising don't work for weight loss, at least if you want to maintain it in the long run.

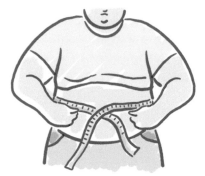

So if cutting calories is not the answer, what is? The next chapter explains the hormonal model for weight loss and how you can use fasting to create a new lower "set weight" for your body.

CHAPTER 5
THE SOLUTION: UNDERSTANDING YOUR HORMONES

If you want to be successful on your weight-loss journey, you need to understand that weight loss and weight gain aren't just a matter of calories in and calories out, something I talk about in Chapter 4. Your weight is influenced by more than the food you eat or how much or little you exercise; weight loss and weight gain are hormonal issues.

The complicated relationship between different hormones in your body decides what your body composition is and how much you weigh. So to lose weight, you need to understand how these hormones work and how you can affect them. I explain that in this chapter.

HOW HORMONES INFLUENCE WEIGHT

Let's first look at how hormones influence weight gain during adolescence. Before puberty, both boys and girls have fairly similar body compositions. They weigh about the same and look about the same. But as they go through puberty, their bodies begin to change; girls start gaining more fat, especially around the hips and thighs, and boys start gaining more muscle.

When this happens, it's not because girls suddenly lose their willpower or that boys suddenly start going to the gym for hours a day. These changes happen completely involuntarily due to hormonal changes, mainly because of increased estrogen for girls and increased testosterone for boys.

Insulin is another key hormone to understand when looking at weight gain and weight loss because the levels of insulin present in your body directly dictate whether your body stores body fat or burns body fat. To put it simply, when insulin levels are high, you gain weight; when insulin levels are low, you lose weight.

One really interesting example showing how insulin affects weight gain and weight loss comes from studying undiagnosed type 1 diabetics. In type 1 diabetes, the body doesn't produce insulin at all, which means one telltale sign of type 1 diabetes before diagnosis is indeliberate and uncontrollable weight loss. People with type 1 diabetes aren't suddenly losing weight because they're eating less or working out more. In fact, you could feed these people almost anything, and they still wouldn't be able to put on weight because their bodies just can't produce the insulin needed to store body fat. However, once these patients are diagnosed and prescribed insulin, they start gaining weight again.

Let me give you another example of how insulin causes weight gain. Insulinomas are rare tumors that constantly release large amounts of insulin into the body, regardless of whether there's glucose present. Because of the constant high levels of insulin, patients with insulinomas gain weight unintentionally, even when they cut calories to try to fight it. Their high levels of insulin cause fat storage and stop the breakdown of stored fat in the body. Once the tumor is removed, patients start to lose weight quickly, even when they keep eating as much as they did before.

Two other hormones can contribute to weight gain:

- If you have high levels of the stress hormone cortisol, you may gain weight, even when you're controlling the number of calories you eat.[1]
- Leptin, which is commonly known as the "fullness hormone," has also been linked to weight gain. Having low levels of leptin can make you feel hungrier, and research has shown that people who have low levels of leptin are more likely to put on weight.[2]

These examples show that weight gain and weight loss is tightly controlled by hormones, not calories. So if you want to lose weight, and more important keep it off, you need to deal with the underlying causes of these hormonal imbalances.

INSULIN RESISTANCE and WHY YOU GAIN WEIGHT DESPITE BEING on a CONSTANT DIET

Insulin resistance happens when the cells in your body become less sensitive to insulin. It causes weight gain, makes it more difficult to lose weight, and is a precursor to developing type 2 diabetes. So if you've been struggling to lose weight for a long time despite trying every diet under the sun, you might be insulin resistant.

What causes insulin resistance? What you eat is the biggest factor. When you eat highly processed foods and carbohydrates such as bread, pasta, and sweet drinks that are quickly broken down into sugar in the bloodstream, your blood glucose levels (and insulin) spike quickly. And when you keep spiking your insulin by constantly snacking and eating a highly processed diet, your body becomes less and less sensitive to insulin, which will eventually "overload" your system. Then, because your cells are less responsive to insulin, your body is forced to release more and more insulin to keep your blood sugar levels under control. It's similar to the way a drug addict needs more and more of their drug to achieve the same effect; your cells need more and more insulin to respond to the blood glucose levels. You now have so much insulin circulating in your blood, with cells that are unable to react to it, that it creates a vicious cycle of more and more insulin but also less and less responsiveness. Eventually, nothing works properly anymore, and your system is completely out of whack.

Traditional "diets" often focus on severely restricting your calories without addressing any of the underlying hormonal imbalances in your body. That's why most so-called diets cause you to gain weight in the long run and may actually make your insulin resistance worse.

When you restrict calories without thinking about the type of calories you're eating, chances are you're still consuming high-carb foods that spike your insulin levels. Most diet foods focus on being "low fat," which usually means they're high in sugar and/or carbs. So even when you're limiting calories, you still have too much insulin in your body, which is what's preventing your body from accessing your stored fat in the first place.

On top of this, when you're a serial dieter, you often lose weight for a period of time only to regain that weight and more later because you're unable to stick to the diet, and you go back to your old eating ways. I used to be guilty of this yo-yo dieting. When you're in this cycle of losing weight and putting it back on several times, your insulin resistance worsens because your body becomes more efficient at storing fat during the nondieting periods to protect itself from future periods of caloric restriction.

High insulin levels can also make you hungrier and more likely to crave high-carb foods, which makes it even more difficult to stick to a calorie-restricted diet in the long run. If you've ever been on a calorie-restricted diet, you probably know that this is true. Eating restrictively eventually leads you to overeat and gain more weight, which only makes the yo-yo dieting cycle worse; in turn, your insulin resistance worsens even more. This is why caloric restriction doesn't actually work.

To finally manage your weight and heal your insulin resistance, you need to lower your insulin levels. You can do this in a few different ways. The number one way to make your body more insulin sensitive is to use intermittent fasting. When you're fasting, you're giving your body a break—periods of time where it's not stimulated to produce any insulin at all because you're not eating anything. When you do this long enough, your high blood insulin levels start to come down, and you eventually become more insulin sensitive as a result.

Another way to heal your insulin resistance is by switching to a low-carb or ketogenic diet. When you stop eating processed carbs and sugars, your insulin levels are lowered. Focus on a diet full of whole, unprocessed foods, fats, and protein to stabilize your blood sugar levels and reduce your body's need for so much insulin. Other ways to lower your insulin levels and achieve sustainable weight loss include doing regular physical exercise, managing your stress levels, and getting enough sleep.

Bottom line: Reducing your insulin levels is key for allowing your body to access and burn your stored body fat. As long as you're insulin resistant, you can't do that, no matter how many diets you go on.

LEPTIN RESISTANCE and WHY YOU'RE CONSTANTLY HUNGRY

Leptin is commonly known as the "fullness hormone," and it's produced from your fat cells. When leptin is released in your body, it reduces your appetite, which in turn helps you manage your weight by signaling you to stop eating.

The general idea is that when you've had enough food and there's enough body fat stored on your body, leptin sends signals to your brain for you to stop being hungry and to stop eating. The more body fat you have, the higher your leptin levels. When your response to leptin works properly, you should be able to maintain a healthy body weight without much effort. Unfortunately, the Western diet has messed this up for many people.

Leptin helps maintain a balanced weight through a feedback loop, like the one shown in Figure 5.1 on the next page.

Figure 5.1
Leptin feedback loop

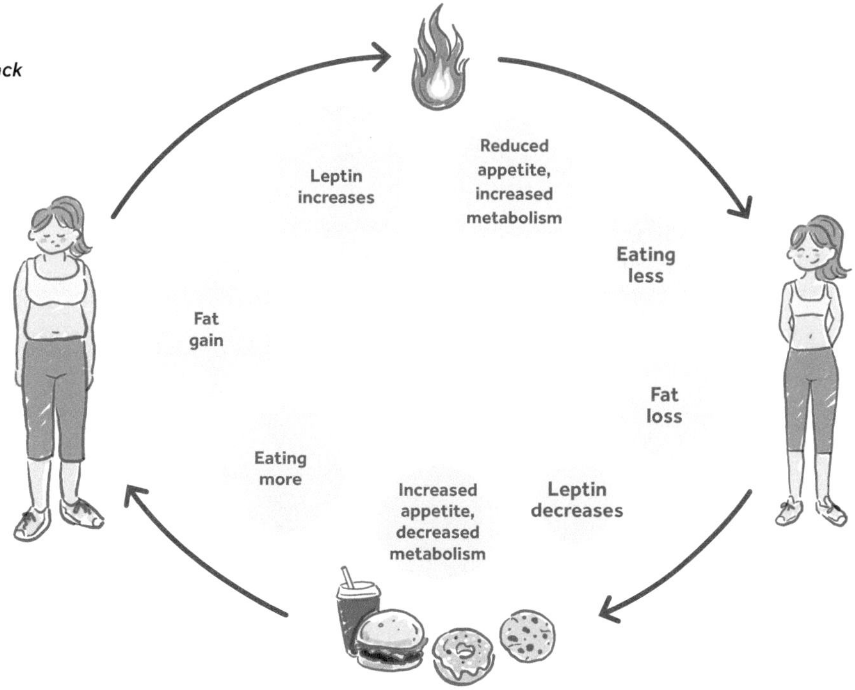

Each time you gain body fat, more leptin is released into your system. More leptin leads to reduced appetite and more energy expenditure because, when there's a lot of leptin circulating in your system, it signals your brain to lower your hunger and lower the amount of food you're eating. It also increases your metabolism, which helps you burn off stored body fat. Each time you lose body fat, less leptin is released into your system, which increases your appetite, so you eat more and gain more body fat.

This feedback loop makes sure that your body weight stays relatively constant over time and works similarly to the way a thermostat maintains an even room temperature.

Leptin resistance is like insulin resistance in that it happens when leptin levels are high, but your body is unable to respond appropriately to it. When you have leptin resistance, your brain doesn't get the proper instructions to reduce appetite and increase energy expenditure. You feel hungry constantly (despite constantly eating); at the same time, you have a lower energy expenditure. In fact, research has confirmed that most obese people are leptin resistant.[3]

There are several reasons why you may develop leptin resistance:

- **High insulin levels:** Having chronically high insulin levels, often because of eating a diet that's high in processed carbs and sugar, disrupts leptin signaling.[4]

- **Inflammation:** Having high levels of inflammation in your body can also disrupt the leptin signaling.[5]

- **Free fatty acids:** When there are too many free fatty acids in your bloodstream, it prevents leptin from being able to send information to your brain.[6]

- **High leptin levels:** Excessively high levels of leptin in your bloodstream make it more difficult for leptin to be absorbed properly.[7]

All these things are usually made worse by obesity, which means it's easy to get stuck in a vicious cycle of gaining weight and becoming more and more leptin resistant over time. (See Figure 5.2.)

The good news is that fasting can help reverse your leptin resistance. When you're fasting, the amount of insulin in your body goes down, which allows leptin to function more effectively. Fasting also reduces the inflammation in your body, which improves leptin signaling in your brain. And finally, fasting helps your body use stored body fat for energy, which reduces the free fatty acid levels in your bloodstream and therefore improves your leptin sensitivity.

Figure 5.2
Leptin and weight-gain cycle

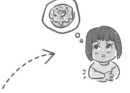

INCREASED CALORIE INTAKE
Even though you increase calorie intake, you are continually hungry, which leads to continued weight gain.

OVEREATING
The brain senses low leptin levels, leading to food cravings and overeating.

WEIGHT GAIN
As you increase fat stores and whole-body inflammation, your body develops leptin resistance.

DISRUPTIVE SIGNAL
Even though you have an abundance of stored fat and leptin, the signal to your brain gets disrupted.

HOW FASTING CAN REDUCE HUNGER

It may seem counterintuitive, but fasting actually makes you feel less hungry. And it's all about how fasting affects your hunger hormones.

Most conventional diets suggest that you should eat several small meals a day to keep your metabolism high and prevent you from getting so hungry you overeat. But thinking that eating frequently makes you less hungry isn't supported by research. One study looked at whether eating breakfast as two small meals would make you less hungry by lunchtime than eating breakfast as one big meal. The study found that people who ate breakfast as two smaller meals were more hungry by lunchtime and had a stronger desire to eat than the people who ate breakfast as one large meal.[8] Another study found that eating more protein made participants feel less hungry, but eating frequent meals did not.[9]

Ghrelin is what's commonly known as the "hunger hormone." It's released to stimulate your hunger and make you want to eat. So to lose weight, you need to know how to control your ghrelin levels.

Some studies have shown that fasting can lower the amount of ghrelin the body produces and therefore can decrease hunger. One study measured participants' ghrelin levels every twenty minutes during a thirty-three-hour fast. It showed that ghrelin (and thus hunger) was highest around the usual mealtimes—breakfast, lunch, and dinner—but also that after the first wave of hunger, ghrelin levels decreased even when the participants didn't eat anything.[10] Another study put participants on an eighty-four-hour fast and found that while ghrelin levels and hunger spiked around mealtimes, overall ghrelin levels decreased the longer the fast went on.[11] That means participants were less hungry despite not eating for three days. This shows that hunger is a learned response that can be triggered in anticipation of food. It also shows that hunger comes and goes in waves and doesn't just get worse and worse over time. If you don't eat anything when the first hunger wave hits, the feeling of needing to eat will eventually go away.

So fasting actually allows you to eat less and feel fuller, which is exactly what you need when you're trying to lose weight.

CORTISOL and WHY STRESS CAN LEAD to WEIGHT GAIN

You might not know it, but stress is a main driver behind weight gain, and if you're chronically stressed, you can seriously be hurting your weight-loss efforts.

Stress causes the release of the hormone cortisol, which is commonly known as the "stress hormone." Research has shown that increased levels of cortisol can lead to weight gain. But why? It comes down to the relationship between cortisol and insulin. Every time you're stressed, your body releases adrenaline with cortisol, which causes glucose to be released into your bloodstream. Your body uses this glucose (or sugar) as a form of quick-release energy to be used in the fight-or-flight response.[12] This was an important response in hunter-gatherer days because it gave people the energy they needed to run away from predators or other threats. When they were scared, cortisol was released, prompting glucose to be released, and they got a burst of energy; they used that energy to run away until they were safe again. So as they dealt with the threat by running or fighting, they burned off the glucose, and adrenaline and cortisol levels normalized.

The problem with modern society is that we don't experience a lot of immediate threats. Instead, we experience loads of chronic stress, including work stress, sleepless nights from taking care of children, and relationship and family stressors. When we're constantly exposed to stress but we don't have a chance to burn off the excess glucose in our blood (because we don't need to run away from anything), we experience constantly high insulin levels because insulin is released to help store the excess glucose in our blood. And as you know, when insulin is high, it prompts your body to store fat.

Evolution is slow, so your body hasn't been able to keep up with the modernization of society. It's impossible for your body to distinguish between a scary work email and a scary tiger that's about to eat you. When you get 100 scary work emails every week and then return home to even more stress due to screaming children or looming deadlines, your cortisol levels are constantly high. But unlike the predators of your hunter-gatherer ancestors, the source of your stress doesn't go away, so the cortisol levels in your body are never allowed to come down long enough to stabilize your blood sugar and insulin. High levels of cortisol unfortunately have a double-whammy effect; they trigger sugar cravings and slow down your metabolism.

The key reason why cortisol triggers sugar cravings is because the quick energy your body needs to run away from a threat can be provided only by carbohydrates. That's also why sugar and carbs are the first things you reach for when you're feeling stressed. The downside to consuming too much sugar, of course, is that your body stores it as fat— particularly in the form of abdominal fat, which can be extra hard to burn off.

So chronic stress leads to a vicious cycle like the one shown in Figure 5.3: You're feeling stressed, so your body releases more cortisol, which makes you crave sugar, which makes you eat more, which makes you gain more and more weight, which makes you feel more and more stressed.

Figure 5.3
Cortisol cycle

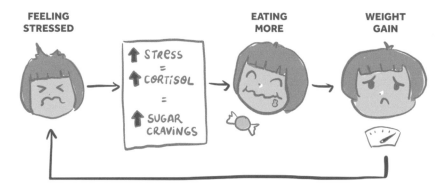

Cortisol not only encourages your body to store fat, but also actively slows down your metabolism, which makes it more difficult for you to lose weight, even if you're not eating high-carb foods. One study found that women who experienced at least one stressor in a period of twenty-four hours burned significantly fewer calories after eating a high-calorie meal compared to women who weren't stressed.[13] The stressed women also had higher levels of insulin than the unstressed women, and, as you know, higher levels of insulin mean more fat storage. When you combine these things, it's clear that they can cause a lot of weight gain over time.

Stress also results in the following situations, which can contribute to weight gain:

- Stress can cause you to engage in unhealthy habits such as emotional eating. When you're stressed, you're more likely to eat for comfort, which means you're more at risk for consuming more calories than you normally would.

- Another complication of stress is that it has been shown to disrupt your sleep patterns. Sleep deprivation has been shown to slow your metabolism and increase your appetite.[14]

Managing your stress levels can help you make sure that you're keeping your hormones balanced and allowing your body to release fat instead of store it.

WEIGHT SET POINT and HOW FASTING CAN RESET IT

Your body has a weight set point, which is basically a weight range where your body is most comfortable. Once your body has settled on a weight set point, it makes a number of adjustments to make sure you go back there even if you gain or lose weight temporarily.

For example, your body can make changes to how hungry you feel, or it can increase or decrease your metabolism. If you overeat, your body increases your body heat so you burn more energy; if you undereat or overexercise, your body increases your hunger so you eat more. Your body makes these adjustments to ensure you stay at your weight set point.

Your weight set point is controlled by a range of different hormones. Insulin (the fat storage hormone), leptin (the fullness hormone), ghrelin (the hunger hormone), and other hormones work together to keep things in check in terms of your energy balance and body weight. When your body weight drops below your weight set point, hunger hormones increase and fullness hormones decrease, which stimulates you to want to eat more. Hormones also reduce the number of calories you burn to help you regain the weight you lost. The same thing happens when you gain. When your weight goes above your body's weight set point, your appetite generally decreases, and your metabolism increases to help you get rid of the extra weight. However, your body is generally better at compensating for weight loss than for weight gain, which is a shame.

So does that mean you'll always stay at the ideal set weight for your body? Unfortunately not. The way we eat and live in modern Western society means that we can damage or completely lose this weight set point regulation. Because you have virtually unlimited access to highly processed and highly palatable foods, it's easy to overeat or to eat for reasons other than hunger. It would be very difficult for you to overeat chicken breast or lettuce, for example. You'd just stop eating when you feel satisfied. But with highly processed foods, you don't have this natural stopping point because these foods have been specifically engineered to light up your brain's reward center, which keeps you wanting more. If you keep overeating and gaining weight above your weight set point, your body eventually settles at a new higher weight set point.

Insulin also plays a part in regulating your weight set point. High levels of insulin can increase your body's weight set point by increasing fat storage and influencing how and when hunger signals are sent to the brain. Obese people often have abnormally high insulin levels as well as a much higher insulin response to food than normal-weight people, which will drive them to gain more weight by increasing the body weight set point.

So is it possible to reset an abnormally high body weight set point? Yes. Fasting can help you reduce your weight set point by lowering insulin levels and improving your insulin sensitivity (healing insulin resistance).

Fasting helps you create a new, lower body weight set point through a few different ways:

- Fasting reduces your insulin levels because you're not eating as often. This allows your body to be in a state of lower insulin longer, which signals your body to burn your stored body fat, in turn helping to lower your weight set point.[15]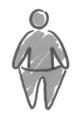

- Fasting improves your insulin sensitivity. A lot of people in modern society are insulin resistant, meaning they're unable to use the insulin produced by the pancreas appropriately to help transport glucose to the cells. This leads to abnormally high levels of blood sugar (and therefore insulin) in the blood, which in turn leads to weight gain. Fasting can help reverse this by improving insulin sensitivity, which means that your body needs less insulin to regulate those blood sugar levels. Improving your insulin sensitivity helps you manage your blood sugar levels more effectively and reduces your body's hormonal drive to store fat.[16]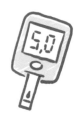

- Fasting influences a number of other important hormones that are involved in hunger and fullness. Counterintuitive as it may sound, fasting actually reduces the hunger hormone ghrelin and increases your sensitivity to the fullness hormone leptin. These two things together will help you feel fuller faster—something that will also help reset your body weight set point.[17]

This chapter explored the complex relationship between hormones and weight changes. While traditional diets reduce weight loss and weight gain to a simple calories-in-versus-calories-out equation, reality is a lot more nuanced. And while fasting can be an excellent tool in helping you manage your weight, there are still a lot of myths and misconceptions around it. In the next chapter, I bust some of the most common fasting myths.

CHAPTER 6
COMMON FASTING MYTHS

There are many myths about fasting. Just tell your friends you're thinking about making fasting part of your life, and you'll likely hear a whole laundry list!

Many of these myths exist simply because people are not educated enough about fasting and its positive effects on the body. In this chapter, I put your mind at ease as I use research to dispel some of the most common fasting myths.

FASTING SLOWS DOWN YOUR METABOLISM

One of the most common myths about fasting is that it'll slow down your metabolism and stop you from losing weight. This couldn't be further from the truth. In fact, research suggests that fasting can improve your metabolism.

Some of the most common diet advice out there is to eat frequent, small meals to keep your metabolism high. However, eating frequently means your insulin levels keep spiking, which is counterproductive to fat loss. To access your stored body fat, you need to keep your insulin levels low. Another form of common weight-loss advice is to restrict your calories, but research has shown that caloric restriction actually leads to a decrease in your metabolism.[1] Fasting, on the other hand, has been shown to increase your metabolism. In fact, fasting for just forty-eight hours can increase your metabolic rate by as much as 14 percent.[2]

How? Well, fasting increases your norepinephrine levels, which stimulates your metabolism and tells your body to break down fat more quickly.[3] Fasting also increases the levels of human growth hormone (HGH) in your body, which helps your body preserve muscle mass and supports a strong metabolism. One study showed that fasting for just two days increases HGH by 500 percent.[4] So, fasting doesn't slow down your metabolism, *and* it makes you burn more fat. Win, win!

FASTING PUTS YOU in "STARVATION MODE"

One of the most common things I hear people say is that fasting will put you in starvation mode, and that's just not true.

Is "starvation mode" real? Yes, there's research to suggest that starvation mode is real and a natural response from your body to protect you against starvation when you experience a dramatic decrease in caloric intake. (The formal term for it is *adaptive thermogenesis*.[5]) The more interesting question is whether fasting puts you in starvation mode.

The key here lies in the difference between fasting and severe caloric restriction. When you're severely restricting your calories through a low-calorie diet, your metabolism slows down so much that it causes you to burn hundreds of calories less every day.[6] This tells us that starvation mode is a real effect, and it also explains why you end up regaining weight after losing weight through caloric restriction.

Because fasting cuts calories completely, people often think that your metabolism will be completely shut down as well. Interestingly, though, when you cut your calories to zero through fasting, your metabolic rate doesn't decrease in the same way that severe caloric restriction decreases it. Because of how fasting affects your hormones, it has a different effect on your metabolism. One study found that while caloric restriction slowed down metabolism, fasting didn't.[7] Other studies have found that fasting actually increases your metabolic rate rather than slows it down.[8] Fasting increases your metabolism and gives you more energy through a few different mechanisms, including increasing your norepinephrine.[9]

And it wouldn't make sense for fasting to put your body into "starvation mode" anyway. Human beings have been going through involuntary periods of fasting for millennia. Our hunter-gatherer ancestors would regularly go days and even weeks without food while they were hunting for animals, and they would need a lot of energy during those times. So if starvation mode from fasting was actually a thing, it would have been very bad for human survival. If our metabolism shut down after only a day without eating, our ancestors would have had a lot less energy to hunt for food, which would have made it more difficult to find food, and that would have shut their metabolism down even more, and so on. So if fasting caused starvation mode, human beings as a species wouldn't have been able to survive. This belief that humans, unlike other animals in the wild, need three to six meals a day to survive just doesn't make sense. In fact, many other mammals go through these fast-and-feast cycles as well. When was the last time you saw an overweight lion? Or a monkey on Weight Watchers? You haven't—because they eat until they're satisfied and then go through periods of fasting.

The easiest way to explain why the idea that fasting causes starvation mode is so unreasonable is to look at an analogy for how you store food in your house. I first heard of this analogy from Dr. Jason Fung, a nephrologist and a strong proponent of fasting, and it's just too good not to share. You have a fridge and a freezer, right? The fridge is where you keep food that you use every day, and the freezer is where you keep food you want to save for later. If you go food shopping three times a day, every day, you'd put some of the groceries straight into the fridge to be eaten in the near future and some of the groceries in the freezer to be eaten later. But if you keep buying food three times a day, quite quickly both your fridge and your freezer will be completely full. If you continue buying more food at that point, you will need to buy more freezers to store all the extra food. As the years go on, you will have to buy more and more freezers to store more and more of the food you don't have time to finish. But if you suddenly stop buying food altogether because you run out of money, you wouldn't starve. Instead, you would finish the food in the fridge before starting to use up all that great stuff in the freezers. With all that stored food, you'd be able to survive for months without shopping.

The same is true for your body. When you eat food, you get quick energy in the form of glucose—which is kind of like the food you have in the fridge. It's easy to access, and you can eat it right away. When you've had enough of what you need for your daily energy, your body turns any extra glucose into body fat so you can use it later—which is kind of like the food in your freezer. If you keep eating, you constantly have plenty of glucose in your body (that is, your fridge is full), which means your body doesn't have a chance to use your body fat (your freezer food) for energy. When you constantly have glucose coming in from eating food, your body fat keeps building up (you buy more and more freezers). But when your glucose levels are running low from fasting, your body doesn't just shut down and put you into starvation mode—it starts to use your stored body fat (or your freezer food) for energy instead.

YOUR BRAIN NEEDS GLUCOSE to FUNCTION

You may have heard that the brain needs glucose to function, and this may be part of why some people are scared to try fasting or a ketogenic diet.

Your brain controls everything in your body and keeps you alive—everything from breathing to keeping you warm and producing hormones. And even though your brain is just 2 percent of your body size, it uses 20 percent of your daily energy needs.[10] Your brain is a pretty important organ, so it's only natural to be concerned.

For your brain to do its job, you need to provide it with energy constantly. That doesn't mean you need to eat constantly, though, because the amazing thing about the brain is that it can use both glucose and ketones for energy. The high-carb diet most people eat ensures that there's always enough glucose available to feed the brain.

But what happens when you keep carbs low or stop eating carbs completely? Will your brain stop working? Not at all. When you're eating a high-carb diet, your brain mainly uses glucose for fuel because there's so much available. But when you're on a low-carb or ketogenic diet, or if you're fasting, your brain instead uses ketones as its main source of energy because there's not a lot of glucose around.[11] Your brain is a really smart cookie.

So how does this process work? When you don't eat carbs for twenty-four to forty-eight hours, the glycogen stores in your liver and muscles run out, meaning your blood sugar and insulin levels drop. At this point, your liver starts to produce ketones, which it makes from breaking down your fat. Ketones can come from the fat you eat or from your body's own fat stores. When there's no glycogen available, these ketones travel into your brain and supply it with a sustainable source of energy.[12]

Although your brain normally uses glucose to function, research has shown that if you're following a strict ketogenic diet, ketones can provide around 70 percent of your brain's energy needs.[13] The remaining glucose your brain needs can be provided by the liver through a process called gluconeogenesis,[14] where your body makes new glucose from proteins, which is why it's important that you eat enough protein on a keto diet.

So, because your brain can get all the energy it needs from either stored glycogen, ketones, or gluconeogenesis, you don't have to eat a high-carb diet to fuel your brain!

FASTING MAKES YOU LOSE MUSCLE

The belief that fasting leads you to lose muscle is another thing that just doesn't make sense. If going a few days without food causes our bodies to burn our muscles for fuel, our ancestors would have ended up weaker and weaker, which would have made them less able to hunt for food. They would eventually have turned into bags of fat and bone and just died.

The question you should ask yourself is this: If our bodies are designed to store energy as body fat, why would it burn our muscles instead? The answer is, of course, that it doesn't. As long as you have enough excess body fat available, your body won't break down your muscles for energy. Muscles are really important! You need your muscles to perform everyday tasks like walking and lifting, and your heart is literally a muscle. It would be seriously disadvantageous for your body to start breaking down your muscles when it has fat stores to use. Your body is very smart, and when you're fasting, it taps into your stored fat for energy while it also protects your lean muscle mass. Using fat as an energy source saves your muscles to make sure you stay strong and healthy.

Research confirms that intermittent fasting helps preserve your muscle mass while promoting fat loss. This is mainly because fasting increases the production of HGH.[15] One study found that alternate-day fasting led to a 6.5 percent reduction in body weight and a 11.4 percent reduction in body fat, but it also showed that there was no change in lean mass (which is your muscle and bone).[16] Another study looked at the one-meal-a-day (OMAD) fasting schedule and found that it caused great levels of fat loss but no signs of muscle loss.[17]

FASTING CAUSES OVEREATING

Another common fasting myth is that it causes overeating. People who are against fasting say that it makes you uncontrollably hungry, which makes you eat more calories as soon as you break your fast. The research doesn't support that viewpoint.

When done carefully and properly, fasting doesn't cause you to overeat. In fact, although studies suggest that fasting might cause a slight increase in the number of calories consumed immediately after breaking your fast, the overall number of calories you eat after fasting still goes down.

One study compared calorie consumption between fasting and nonfasting groups. It was found that if a person normally eats 2,436 calories a day, they consumed slightly more calories after fasting (2,914 calories). But when you look at the results over the course of two days, those who fasted consumed 1,958 calories less than those who didn't fast.[18] In other words, eating slightly more right after fasting doesn't cancel out the fasting benefits.

Another key here is mindset. How you think about fasting affects your likelihood of overeating. If you see fasting as punishment or deprivation, you could end up eating too much after breaking your fast. Fasting should always be approached from a calm and centered mindset. It has many benefits for your health and isn't all about weight loss, and it's not about deprivation. So if you approach fasting with a proper mindset and remember all the good things you're doing for your body, you're much less likely to overeat after breaking your fast.

FASTING MAKES YOU UNCONTROLLABLY HUNGRY

When you're fasting, you will feel hungry sometimes; that's just part of it. But does it really make you feel *hungrier*? Not really. Hunger during fasting is a lot less of a problem than you might think.

The important thing is to understand how fasting affects the hormone ghrelin, which is your body's "hunger hormone." When ghrelin is released in your body, it makes you feel hungry. So to lose weight, it only makes sense that you try to decrease the amount of ghrelin you have in your body. That's exactly what fasting does!

Studies have shown that ghrelin is actually lowest first thing in the morning.[19] Now, if hunger truly was about the number of hours you've gone without food, you should be the *most* hungry in the morning because you haven't eaten for eight or more hours. But most people are not that hungry in the morning because hunger is a hormonal response that has very little to do with how long you've gone without food. In fact, one study showed that during a three-day fast, hunger gradually decreased the longer the fast went on.[20]

The reason hunger decreases during a fast is because fasting changes the way hunger hormones are released in your body. Studies have found that fasting reduces ghrelin, making you feel less hungry.[21] One twenty-four-hour fasting study looked at fasting's effect on ghrelin levels and found some interesting patterns. The study didn't find that ghrelin continued to rise the longer the participants fasted. Instead, it found that ghrelin levels, and therefore hunger, spiked during the times when the participants would normally expect to eat (such as at breakfast, lunch, and dinner) but decreased overall with time.[22] This suggests that hunger is a somewhat learned response based on your daily habits. It also shows that hunger comes and goes in waves and doesn't just get worse and worse. If you ride those hunger waves, the hunger will gradually decrease even if you don't eat.

Another study showed that intermittent fasting not only reduced ghrelin but also increased fullness and decreased the desire to eat.[23] In other words, fasting can make you feel less hungry on the whole and doesn't automatically cause more hunger, as many people think it does.

Now that you know about the history and science behind fasting, let's move onto fasting in practice. In the following section of the book, I walk you through the practical steps for how you can use fasting to transform your health, including sections on mindset and motivation, diet, and managing potential side effects. The next chapter covers the twelve fundamentals to fasting for weight loss.

2

THE HOW OF FASTING

CHAPTER 7

THE 12 FUNDAMENTALS OF FASTING FOR WEIGHT LOSS

Fasting can be confusing. There are many different voices talking about fasting, and the volume of information can be overwhelming.

To help you be as successful as possible on your fasting journey, I have put together a list of my twelve fundamentals of fasting for weight loss. By following these simple rules, you'll be able to transform your health and weight in no time.

BE CLEAR ABOUT YOUR WHYS

When you're fasting, one of the most important things you need when you start is an understanding of your whys, which is a list of the reasons you're fasting, and why you're on this journey. Your whys can range from everything from weight loss to feeling better in your own skin to getting healthier or preventing diseases such as type 2 diabetes. Whatever your reasons, be as clear and specific about them as you can.

Write all of your whys down. Writing your whys on a piece of paper is better than typing them on your phone or computer because you give yourself a greater chance to absorb things when you physically write them. You want to give yourself the best chance to internalize your whys so you can manifest them and start living them.

Divide your list of whys into short-term whys and long-term whys. Short-term whys could be wanting to look good for a specific event or an upcoming birthday or fitting into a specific piece of clothing. Long-term whys tend to be more focused on health and family, such as wanting to live longer so you can be there for your kids and grandkids or preventing yourself from developing obesity-related conditions like type 2 diabetes or heart disease. Think about reasons that are personal and specific to you and your circumstances. Give as much detail as you can, and then keep your list of whys with you and read it every day.

As you advance on this journey, your whys might change, or you might feel the need to add more. Add to your list of whys as you progress and learn more about yourself.

Throughout this journey, you're going to have to remind yourself of your whys many times, especially when you hit moments of weakness or when you're struggling with motivation. So keeping your list of whys at the front and center every single day is going to make your journey easier and more manageable.

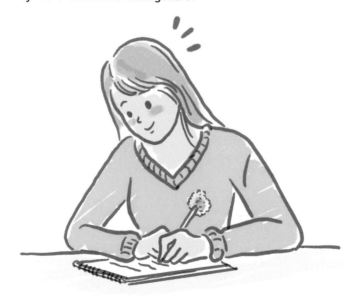

KNOW YOUR EXCUSES

The next task is to make a list of your excuses. Again, I want you to take a pen and a piece of paper and write them all down.

Record everything you can think of that you tell yourself whenever you've fasted or tried to lose weight in the past—all the excuses or reasons to go off track or break your fast. Also try to imagine some excuses that you think you might tell yourself, even if you've never used them before. The excuses can be big or small, but they're all part of the mind games that you may play on yourself as you progress through this journey. By making a list of your excuses, you're "calling them out" and taking their power away, which is the first step in beating them.

Sample excuses are things like

- This is too difficult.
- I will never reach my goal weight anyway, so I might as well stop.
- I can just try calorie counting instead.

If you're really honest with yourself and go deep, your list of excuses can end up being quite lengthy. That's a good thing because you're going to keep the list and read it to yourself every single day. It's especially important to read it in the moments when you're struggling because chances are good that you'll be telling yourself one or several of these excuses in those weak moments. When you've anticipated your thoughts and you have them on that list, you're able to identify them as excuses rather than mistaking them for real reasons to break your fast or go off track. Your list of excuses is an extra obstacle or a shield against your own mind trickery.

JOIN a SUPPORT GROUP

One of the best things you can do on your fasting journey is to get support from other people who are going through the same thing as you.

There are many different support groups out there, and many of them are online and global, which is amazing because they give you round-the-clock access to support.

Joining a support group is a great way to feel like you're not going through this alone. A lot of times, people around you might not be fasting, or they might not be supportive of your journey, so surrounding yourself (even digitally) with people who are supportive and who are going through the same thing can make a world of difference.

A support group also provides you with the hive mind—the collective knowledge of thousands of people who have fasted for hundreds and thousands of hours and who have likely gone through all of the struggles that you're facing. People in the group will be able to provide you with knowledge, resources, and experience from their journeys, and you'll be able to return the favor by providing your own knowledge, support, and resources to others. Online support groups have been instrumental on my own journey to fast myself fit.

MOVE DAILY

Getting out and moving daily is another fundamental on your fasting journey. You don't have to go to the gym every day or do blisteringly fast cardio or high-intensity interval training (HIIT).

In fact, you're better off not doing intense exercise because it can increase your stress levels and hurt your weight-loss efforts. Daily movement can be as simple as going for a walk.

On my own weight-loss journey, I didn't step foot in the gym a single time, but I did go for daily one-hour walks. Walks are great because they do more than get your body moving; they also get your mind moving. Walking every day can help you stay motivated and keep your mind clear and focused. Whenever you find yourself struggling with mind games or going through a rough patch, just put on your walking shoes and head outside. Walking can be incredibly therapeutic for the mind, and it can help keep your stress levels down (which is another key to fasting success).

KEEP YOUR STRESS LEVELS DOWN

Stress in small doses is usually nothing you have to be too concerned about. It's a normal response in the body. But chronic or prolonged stress can have really damaging effects on both your physical and mental health.

As I've mentioned in other chapters, stress causes the release of cortisol and adrenaline as part of the fight-or-flight response. The reason this response exists is to provide you with energy quickly when you're presented with a threat, and it goes back to our hunter-gatherer days when our ancestors would frequently have to fight or run away from dangerous animals. To deal with such threats, we needed adrenaline to get our energy levels up, and cortisol to release sugar into our bloodstream quickly. Once we'd dealt with the threat, adrenaline levels could go down, and eventually, so would cortisol. But in modern society, our stressors tend not only to be acute but also chronic, and that's where things get tricky.

Stressors from work, relationships, financial worries, and family dynamics contribute to a constant high level of stress in most people's lives. When the stress level is constantly high, you don't experience that natural decrease in adrenaline and cortisol after a stressful event. Instead, your stress hormones stay elevated, which can affect your body, your thoughts, your feelings, and your behavior.

Research has shown that increased cortisol levels can increase your cravings for carbs and sugary foods.[1] You usually crave sugar in these situations because sugar gives your body the quick energy it needs when it thinks there's a threat nearby. The downside to this in modern society is that when you're not fighting a dangerous animal or running away from a dangerous situation, you don't burn off the excess sugar in the bloodstream. Instead, it gets converted into body fat. On top of that, if you eat extra snacks from craving sugar, you store even more fat.

So, what can you do to manage your stress levels? Start to deal with the underlying causes of the stress in your life. Improve your work-life balance, work on your relationships, and ask for support when you need it.

By managing your stress levels, you can break free from the cycle of increased cortisol, insulin spikes, and fat storage. Gaining weight through stress is not about willpower or self-control. It's a physiological response. When you know that, you can manage it more easily. Lower your stress levels by journaling, meditating, going for a walk, or doing breathing exercises.

Journaling

One of the best ways to keep your mind healthy is to journal. Journaling helps you reflect on the thoughts and feelings that are going on in your mind. When you're going through a stressful time, sometimes writing or talking about the situation helps, and putting things down on paper can work as a form of self-therapy. Look for guided journaling topics online or just write whatever comes to your mind.

Meditation

Another great way to keep your stress levels down is to meditate. You don't have to do an hour-long retreat-style mental exercise. You can simply take three to five minutes at the beginning of each day to sit down on the floor to properly ground yourself, close your eyes, and count your breaths in and out. Every time you find your mind wandering, begin your counting again. The more you practice, the further you'll get in your counting, and the lower your stress levels will be.

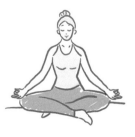

Going for Walks

Another one of my favorite ways to beat stress is to go for daily walks. Walks are not only good for keeping your body moving; they're great for keeping your mind moving too. I often find that I solve problems and calm my racing mind when I go for walks. Getting fresh air, getting some sunlight on your skin, and moving your body forward can make a huge difference for your mental state. I recommend going for walks in silence so you can listen to the sounds of nature. Listening to music or podcasts doesn't allow you to fully connect with yourself and lower your stress.

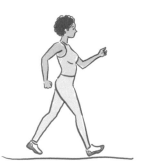

Breathing Exercises

Finally, breathing exercises are an excellent tool for lowering your stress levels. There are many different breathing exercises, but one of my favorite ones is box breathing. The basics of box breathing are that you close your eyes and breathe in for four counts, hold for four counts, breathe out for four counts, and hold for four counts. You repeat this pattern of breathing for a few minutes or until you feel like your mind has calmed. Box breathing is a great exercise when you're in an acutely stressful situation and you need a way to calm yourself quickly.

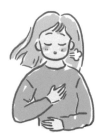

FOLLOW a LOW-CARB DIET

If you want to lose the most amount of weight in the shortest amount of time, I recommend that you combine fasting with a ketogenic diet.

Of course, you can lose weight while fasting and not following a low-carb or ketogenic diet, but that's just making it unnecessarily hard for yourself. Fasting can already be a challenge, so why make it more difficult?

Following a ketogenic diet while fasting not only makes fasting easier because it makes you less hungry, but it also supercharges your fat loss. This is because a ketogenic diet puts you in ketosis, which is the same metabolic state induced through fasting, and it's the process where your body breaks down your stored body fat for fuel. So when you're using a ketogenic diet with fasting, you're supercharging that state of ketosis because you'll be in ketosis when you're fasting as well as when you're not fasting. And that's how you get the pounds moving quickly.

NO "EATING WINDOWS"

When most people think about intermittent fasting, they think about a fasting window and an eating window. For example, you might have a sixteen-hour fasting window and an eight-hour eating window, as with the 16:8 intermittent fasting schedule.

The trouble many people get into with this way of thinking is that they fast for sixteen hours and then eat as many meals as they want during the eight-hour eating window. This is a bad idea because it keeps your insulin levels constantly elevated during the eight-hour period. And because insulin levels are kept high when you're constantly eating or grazing, you'll struggle to lose weight if you approach intermittent fasting this way. That's why I don't recommend an "eating window," as such.

Instead, you should fast for sixteen hours and eat the same number of meals you would normally eat within the remaining eight-hour time period. On a 16:8 intermittent fasting schedule, that would usually mean skipping breakfast and having only lunch and dinner. You would have lunch at around 12:00 p.m. and dinner by 7:00 p.m., finishing your meal before 8:00 p.m. No snacking or grazing between the two meals, and eat your meal in only as much time as you need to finish it. This ensures that you keep your insulin levels as low as possible, and you give your body enough of a break to digest your food and lower your insulin levels.

NO SNACKING BETWEEN MEALS

The previous fundamental of no eating windows ties into no snacking between meals. When you're fasting, the most important thing to remember is that you're trying to keep insulin levels low for as long as possible. And you keep insulin levels low by not eating.

Common dietary advice says to eat three meals a day and throw two or three snacks in there as well. But eating like this keeps your insulin levels high, which means you're constantly storing body fat. When you're intermittent fasting, you cut down on the number of times you eat per day, which means you also cut down on the number of insulin spikes. So stay away from snacking—there is absolutely no need for it. Whatever intermittent fasting schedule you're on, make sure you're only eating the meals associated with that schedule, and don't snack between those meals.

NEVER EAT if YOU'RE NOT HUNGRY

If you're not used to fasting, you might be scared of hunger. Hunger is a natural response that the human body has developed through millions of years of evolution in order to motivate you to start finding food.

In modern society, of course, we don't have to hunt for food; most people just need to open a cupboard or the refrigerator door to find an abundance of it. Consequently, if we act on every single hunger pang, we'd end up gaining weight uncontrollably, which is something a lot of people around the world are struggling with today.

The other side of the coin is that a lot of people are scared not to eat even if they're not hungry. A lot of us have been bombarded with messages about how often we need to eat—for example, that we need to eat constantly to keep our metabolism high, or that we need to eat breakfast regardless of whether we're hungry because breakfast is the most important meal of the day. This is simply not true. When you're fasting, you'll teach your body to burn your stored body fat for energy, and you'll start to tune in to your true hunger and fullness cues. But it's up to you to actually start listening to those cues. If you get to the end of your fasting window and you find that you're not hungry yet, don't eat. Your body is telling you that it's doing fine and it doesn't need food right now, so you can calmly wait. As long as you have enough stored body fat, your body has all the energy it needs. So if you're not hungry in your eating window, just see it as an opportunity to extend your fast a little further.

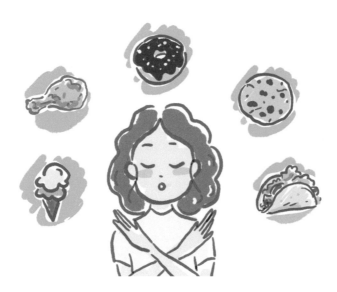

ONLY EAT UNTIL YOU'RE SATISFIED

Part of learning about your body's true hunger and fullness cues is knowing when to stop eating.

The way we eat in modern society—with highly processed foods—leads lot of people to be prone to overeating. Human physiology is not made to process these highly addictive and highly palatable foods, and so we very easily overeat on them. This leads to increased insulin levels, which over time lead to increased insulin resistance and weight gain in a self-perpetuating cycle. So when you're retraining your body to listen to your fullness cues by using fasting and a low-carb diet, it's important that you stop eating at the point when you feel satisfied but not stuffed.

Many people think that they're eating until they're full, but they're actually eating to the point of being stuffed, which is when you feel like you couldn't possibly fit another bite in your mouth. This feeling actually means you're taking your fullness too far. Eating until you're satisfied is different from this, and it's quite a neutral feeling. You're at the point where you're just not hungry anymore but no more full than that.

Use mindful eating to check in with yourself during your meals and ask yourself if you're still hungry. If you're not, and you feel a neutral, satisfied feeling, that's your cue to stop eating. Learning to eat this way will make you feel a lot calmer around food, and it'll make it much easier for you to manage your weight.

Note that you should stop eating *even if there's still food left on your plate.* "But, Emma! The horror! How could you say such a thing?!" During childhood, a lot of us were told, "Finish what's on your plate!" but I'm here to give you permission not to. Of course, I recommend that you try not to put more food on your plate than what you think you can finish, but if you've eaten enough to feel satisfied, you need to get comfortable with leaving food behind. Whether there's half a plate of food left or just *one bite*—leave it. Don't force yourself to finish food because "it's a shame to waste it." I'm telling you the food is already wasted, and it won't do any more good at the bottom of your stomach than it will in the fridge (if you can save it for later) or in the trash (if you can't save it for later). Either you can put the food scraps in the trash or you can treat *yourself* like trash. Your choice.

TAKE YOUR ELECTROLYTES

You should always supplement with electrolytes when you're fasting, especially if you're fasting for twenty-four hours or more.

When you're fasting and following a ketogenic diet, you're losing a lot of fat, but you're also losing water weight. When you're losing water, you're flushing out some important minerals, and you can feel unwell as a result. By taking sodium, magnesium, and potassium every day, you avoid unpleasant side effects like headaches, nausea, and weakness.

The easiest way to take your electrolytes is through an electrolyte supplement; I recommend finding one in pill form. You can take them in powder form as well, but that usually means spending your days drinking salty water, which isn't the most pleasant thing. Also, be aware that most electrolyte supplements on the market contain sweeteners (which are not safe for fasting and will break your fast) and usually don't contain nearly enough of everything you need.

Check out the following table for the daily electrolyte requirements when you're fasting. For intermittent fasting, you should stay on the lower end of the daily requirements; for extended fasting, you should be on the higher end. The supplementation amounts listed are in addition to what you receive from dietary sources on a keto diet. There are many brands of electrolytes available for purchase; make sure you check that they contain enough of each of electrolytes and they are completely free of sweeteners or flavorings.

Electrolytes	Daily requirements	DIY recipe
Sodium (Na)	5,000–7,000 mg/day	3 teaspoons of sea salt or Himalayan salt
Magnesium (Mg)	300–500 mg/day	There are many brands of magnesium supplements. Capsules are easier for many people to swallow than tablets. Choose one that has approximately 500 mg of magnesium.
Potassium (K)	1,000–3,500 mg/day	½ to 1½ teaspoons of potassium citrate powder provide approximately 1,000 to 3,000 mg of potassium. 1 teaspoon of potassium chloride (NuSalt) will provide 3,180 mg of potassium.

STICK to the APPROVED FASTING LIQUIDS

The last fundamental is that you need to stick to the approved fasting liquids. As a general rule, you can only have water, black coffee, and plain tea when you're fasting. These are the three beverages that will serve you best whether you're on an intermittent fast or an extended fast.

Stay away from energy drinks, diet sodas, or flavored waters. You also can't have any juices, smoothies, protein shakes, collagen drinks, or other things like that.

If you can't get by with only water, black coffee, and plain tea, there are a few other approved fasting liquids, but you should use them only as a crutch and only when you're doing an extended fast (a fast longer than forty-eight hours). Examples of these approved bonus fasting liquids are heavy cream, MCT oil, butter, unsweetened pickle juice, and bone broth. For these additional liquids, you're allowed 1 to 2 tablespoons in up to 6 cups of coffee or tea a day, or 1 to 2 tablespoons of bone broth or pickle juice up to six times a day. So it doesn't mean you can drink several cups of pickle juice or bone broth; only have very small sips, and only in situations where you're really struggling and you're very close to breaking your fast if you don't use a crutch. Using approved fasting liquids as a crutch is a great way to extend your fast a little bit longer.

Approved Fasting Lliquids

NOTE

The additional approved fasting liquids are only approved if you're fasting for weight loss. If you're fasting for autophagy, you can have only water, black coffee, and plain tea.

| Water (plain or sparkling) | Black coffee | Tea (black, green or herbal) |

For an Extended Fast

Plus 1-2 tablespoons of any of the following in up to 6 cups of coffee or tea per day

Pickle juice   Bone broth   Heavy cream   Butter   MCT oil   Coconut oil

CHAPTER 8
YOUR FASTING BLUEPRINT

If you're completely new to fasting, not eating for several hours or days can seem daunting. But as long as you start small and keep practicing, you'll soon find it's the easiest thing you've ever done for weight loss. In this chapter, I outline what you need to know to start fasting and be successful on your weight-loss journey.

GETTING STARTED with FASTING

I recommend introducing a ketogenic diet before you get into fasting and especially before you get into longer fasts (such as thirty-six hours or longer). The keto diet is high in fats and very low in carbohydrates, so fasting and the keto diet work well together because both promote ketosis, where you force your body to use your stored body fat instead of food for energy.

When you switch to a ketogenic diet before you start fasting, the transition into fasting can be much smoother because your body is already accustomed to ketosis. A keto diet also makes you feel less hungry, which makes fasting a lot more comfortable. Also, combining fasting with keto increases the health benefits, which include improved insulin sensitivity and more weight loss. You can read more about the keto diet and how to get started in Chapter 13.

When you're ready to start fasting, if you've never tried it before, I recommend starting with a simple schedule, such as 16:8. The 16:8 fasting schedule, when you fast for sixteen hours and eat your meals within an eight-hour window, is a really good starting point for beginners. The easiest way to think about this schedule is to skip breakfast and have lunch and dinner.

What a lot of people get wrong with the 16:8 schedule is eating too much in the eight-hour window. They eat lunch, snacks, dinner, and then more snacks. But having three or six meals within the eight-hour eating window is a mistake that can potentially lead to a lot of weight gain, and it prevents you from getting the most benefits out of fasting. So my suggestion is to stick to just two meals within your eight-hour eating window, with no snacks at all.

The 16:8 schedule easily fits into most lifestyles because you can complete most of your fasting hours while you sleep. Let's say that you finish dinner at 8:00 p.m. and skip breakfast the next morning, waiting until noon to have your first meal. You've just done a sixteen-hour fast with very little effort!

The 16:8 schedule is easy to start and adjust to your daily life; it causes as little disruption as possible. It's easy to keep having lunch with your colleagues and dinner with your family in the evening, and you can easily adapt it to the hours that work for you, meaning you can personalize your eating window to match your routine. If you need to have dinner with your family at 7:00 p.m., you can have your lunch at 11:00 a.m. Finally, the 16:8 schedule is a gentle introduction to fasting and getting your body used to longer fasting hours.

Here are a few tips for fasting correctly:

- **Make sure you hydrate.** Water, black coffee, and plain tea are all great, and none of them will break your fast as long as you don't add anything to them like sugar, honey, milk, or lemon.

- **Stay on top of your electrolytes.** To avoid unpleasant side effects like headaches or nausea, you need to make sure that you keep your electrolytes balanced, especially if you're going for longer fasts. The best and easiest way to get enough electrolytes is to take an electrolyte supplement that contains sodium, magnesium, and potassium. Read more about supplementing with electrolytes in Chapter 7.

- **Break your fast with a low-carb meal.** When it's time to break your fast, eat a light low-carb meal that's easy to digest—for example, salmon with cauliflower. If you eat a heavy meal immediately after fasting, it can make you uncomfortable and result in digestive issues.

- **Always listen to your body.** Some discomfort during fasting is normal and to be expected, but if you experience extreme adverse side effects, such as fainting or throwing up, they're a sign that you're not fasting correctly, and you need to break your fast. If you experience extreme side effects, make sure you reevaluate your fasting schedule and talk to your doctor.

- **Stay consistent.** Change takes time, and staying consistent is key if you want to reach your goal weight. Feeling some hunger is totally OK, and your cravings and hunger will go down as you get accustomed to fasting. The key is not to give up at the first sign of weakness. Push through it: You'll get stronger, and fasting will get easier. Each step of the way, you're building your fasting muscle.

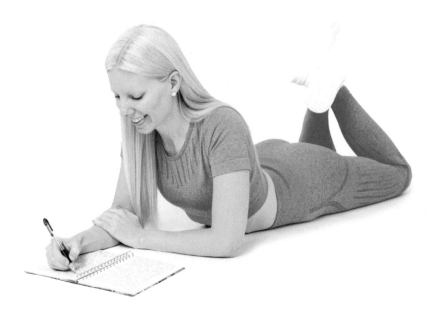

FIGURING OUT WHAT WORKS for YOU

Fasting is not a one-size-fits-all situation. To be successful, you need to adapt your fasting schedule so it fits best with your work-life balance and lines up with your personal health and weight-loss goals. You'll likely have to go through a lot of trial and error before you get really good at fasting, and you have to learn how to listen to and manage your body's cues and signals.

Picking Your Fasting Plan

Think about your daily schedule and try to identify periods when fasting would be most manageable. For example, if you usually have a really busy morning routine, you might be better off skipping breakfast than trying to eat in the morning and fasting for the rest of the day.

You should also think about how your fasting schedule fits around your work schedule. If you have a very physically demanding job, you might find it easier to start with shorter fasts to help your body get used to it. I find that fasting is easier when I'm busy because I have less time to think about food and hunger. In fact, one of the longest fasts I did was a seven-day fast during a week when I was busy baking a wedding cake. Before I became a fasting coach, I dabbled in the cake-making business. One summer, I had a wedding cake due for a Saturday wedding in the south of England. I took this as an opportunity to fast for the whole week leading up to the wedding, and it was actually a lot easier than I thought it was going to be. Baking and decorating the cake took six twelve-hour days of work. Being around all the sugar and flour didn't bother me that much, and being so busy trying to hit the deadline helped keep my mind off food. I wasn't really hungry for the six days I was working on the cake. By the time I delivered the cake, it had been seven days since my last meal. To this day, that's the easiest extended fast I've ever done. If work is also a distraction for you, having a busy or physically demanding job can be a positive that helps you fast for a longer period.

Also consider any family and social commitments. If you have dinner with your family every night, OMAD might be the best fasting plan for you because you can fast while still being able to enjoy evening dinners with your family. But you can also make tweaks to your normal routine if you want to fast longer. For example, if you're usually the person who cooks, you can ask someone else to cook some nights, or you can cook for your family but not participate in eating every night. You can still sit at the table and enjoy a nice hot cup of herbal tea and have good conversations while everyone else is eating. Having a cup of tea or coffee when you need to be around others who are eating is a great way to keep your hands occupied and get something nice and hot in your belly.

What works for others might not work for you, and vice versa, so take some time to figure out your optimal schedule. Finding a fasting schedule that's comfortable but challenging enough to push you to where you want to be ensures you reach your goals while still finding time for friend and family commitments.

Setting Realistic Goals

It's also important to set realistic goals for yourself on your fasting journey. When I first started my journey, I had really high energy, which made me set goals that were too aggressive. For example, I tried to do a three-day fast without doing any research at all. I wanted quick results, so I pushed too hard and was too ambitious. I failed so many times, and not being able to keep up with my goals made me feel down and frustrated.

Keep your goals realistic. Instead of using general statements such as, "I want to get fit," make specific and measurable goals such as, "I will do 16:8 for seven days in a row," or, if you're a more experienced faster, "I will complete a full week of keto OMAD." It's better to set small goals that you actually achieve than aggressive goals that set you up for failure. Positive momentum is a powerful motivator, and negative momentum can completely ruin your chance of success. Once you have smaller accomplishments like these under your belt, you'll feel more confident and motivated, and it will help you build positive momentum.

After you're comfortable with shorter fasts, push yourself to fast a bit longer. Try a twenty-four- or forty-eight-hour fast and then extend your fasting hours from there. As a general rule, the longer you fast, the more weight you'll lose, but you need to find a balance between what you want to do and what you realistically can do. Your goals should push you, but they shouldn't break you. You should aim to go past your comfort zone, but you shouldn't overwhelm and demotivate yourself in the process because you'll risk not reaching your goals at all. If you've never done a fast before, a goal of doing a seven-day fast or losing 30 pounds in a month is too ambitious, and it's not realistic for you to make that your first target. Rome wasn't built in a day, and you're not going to lose all your weight overnight. It's better to start with something you're more likely to achieve, like one successful sixteen- or twenty-four-hour fast, and then build up your confidence from there. *The best fast is the one you can stick to.*

Also make sure that you focus on the *journey* and not just the end goal. Enjoy reaching your short-term goals and improving yourself; then celebrate when you hit a milestone—like losing your first pound or getting through your first twenty-four-hour fast. Doing my first forty-eight-hour fast was huge for me, and I felt superhuman. A two-day fast might seem like a minor achievement to others, but it was the longest fast I'd ever done and represented a massive step on my journey. Progress, however small it may seem, keeps you moving forward.

You also need to be flexible. Life comes with many unexpected situations, and you'll have times when fasting just isn't possible. In these situations, you should adapt your goals without feeling guilty about it. For example, imagine you committed to a twenty-four-hour fast but your boss schedules an important client meeting at lunch. In this case, you can change your fasting goal to fit the situation. Fasting to get fit is a marathon, not a sprint, and sometimes you need to be flexible in the short run to get results in the long run.

WALKING THROUGH a TYPICAL FASTING DAY

To help give you an idea of what a fasting day might look like, in this section, I run through how I manage the day on the two most common schedules: 16:8 and one meal a day (OMAD). How you structure your day is completely up to you. The schedules I include here are just examples of how a typical fasting day might go.

The 16:8 Schedule

On a typical 16:8 day, I start with a glass of water and my electrolyte supplements. Remember, on a 16:8 day, you typically don't eat breakfast. So for the first few hours, I drink only water, but you can have black coffee or plain tea. Don't add anything to your coffee or tea; milk, sweeteners, or other additives break your fast.

In the morning of a 16:8 fasting schedule, I usually like to go for a long walk, aiming for roughly an hour. Going for a walk in the morning helps wake your body up, and it also allows you to clear your mind for the day ahead. I also journal on most days because the morning is a good time to get some thoughts down on paper. I read my list of whys to set my goals for the day.

I usually aim to break my fast around noon. About thirty minutes before breaking my fast, I have a large glass of water mixed with apple cider vinegar to prepare my body for breaking the fast, and I take a fiber supplement. Read more in Chapter 12 about how breaking your fast with fiber and acid can supercharge weight loss. I like to break my fast with a low-carb meal such as eggs and bacon with avocado, or scrambled eggs with smoked salmon. You can have any keto meal you'd like—just make sure that you eat only until you're satisfied, not stuffed. I usually finish my meal with another large glass of water.

After my first meal, I only drink water until it's time for my next meal around 7:00 p.m. Don't have any snacks between your two meals, but you're allowed to drink water, black coffee, or plain tea. The aim here is to get your insulin levels as low as possible between your meals.

My evening meal is another keto meal, such as steak with broccoli and sautéed mushrooms, or salmon with asparagus and avocado. Again, I recommend that you take a glass of water mixed with apple cider vinegar and a fiber supplement about thirty minutes before your meal, and finish with a glass of water to signal the end of the meal. You don't need to count any calories—just eat your one meal for as long as it takes you to finish it (usually no more than twenty minutes), and stop eating when you feel satisfied but not stuffed.

After this meal, I don't have anything else to eat until lunchtime the next day, and I stick to plain water or herbal tea in the evening.

OMAD Schedule

On the OMAD schedule, I approach my day very similarly to a 16:8 day, but instead of breaking my fast at noon, I push through and have my one meal by breaking my fast at 7:00 p.m. I usually start my day off with a glass of water and electrolytes, and I always drink plenty of water and herbal tea throughout the day. Again, you can have only water, black coffee, and plain tea during this twenty-four-hour fasting period. Don't add anything to your drinks, and don't snack. Fasting means you eat nothing at all.

I recommend going for a walk during your fasting period and also journaling and meditating to keep your mind as calm as possible. It's also important to remember that you'll feel hungry during a twenty-four-hour fast, which is completely normal and nothing to be worried or scared about. Hunger is a natural response in your body, and it won't harm you. Hunger comes and goes in waves, so you just have to ride the wave until it passes after a little while. Make sure you keep yourself busy, and keep drinking water to help calm the hunger pangs.

As you approach 7:00 p.m., get your body ready to break your fast by having a glass of water mixed with apple cider vinegar and a fiber supplement. I recommend doing this around thirty minutes before your meal. To break my fast, I have a keto meal such as chicken thighs with asparagus, or fish with a green side salad. I suggest you keep any keto meals as simple as possible—pick a meat, a green vegetable, and a fat—and stay away from processed foods.

Once again, make sure you eat only until you're satisfied, not stuffed, and finish your meal with a glass of water. After your evening meal, you won't have another meal until the following evening at around 7:00 p.m., meaning that you will have fasted for twenty-three to twenty-four hours.

MAINTAINING CONSISTENCY and PROGRESS

To be successful with fasting and losing weight, you need to make sure that you're consistent and that you build a good routine.

Every fast is different—some days will be hard and others will be easier—but no matter what happens, you should try to stay as committed and consistent as possible.

It's important that you stick to your fasting schedule once you choose it. Don't keep setting and rearranging your schedule every few days or hours. To get stronger and better at fasting, you need to build your confidence and trust in yourself.

You should also prepare what you're going to eat to break your fast before you start. You don't have to cook it in advance, but you should at least have the ingredients at home and know what you're having. Being prepared helps you avoid making impulsive decisions that take you away from your goals.

Being consistent also means pushing through hard times. I can't tell you the number of times I've wanted to quit because my fast was getting difficult or I was getting too hungry. But every time I gave up, I wished I had pushed through; and every time I managed to push through, I felt so much better afterward. Each time you push through a hard time, you'll get stronger and better at it the next time.

At the same time, please forgive yourself if you do end up breaking early. Accept it, learn from it, and then move on. Building consistency is about picking yourself up and quickly getting back in the race, so don't dwell on the negatives, and just start again.

It's also important to track your progress and trust the process. Tracking your progress can be incredibly motivating. Use a journal or a tracking app to record your fasting hours, meals, feelings, and your weight and measurements. When you track, you can objectively measure your progress even when you don't feel like you're making any. There will be days when the scale doesn't budge or you feel like all your efforts are for nothing. At those times, it's important to remember that progress happens in a lot of different ways. Sometimes you might not have lost any weight on the scale, but you might have lost inches around your body, your clothes might fit better, or you might have been able to fast for longer periods this week. Trust in the fasting process and know that every step forward is a step toward what you want to achieve.

BUILDING YOUR FASTING MUSCLE

Starting a fasting journey is almost like going to the gym for the first time. In the beginning, you're probably pretty weak, and you don't have the correct form. But the same way your muscles get stronger every time you lift weights, your fasting muscle gets stronger every time you successfully complete a fast or push through a hard time.

Fasting is a skill, and just like any other skill, it requires consistency and discipline so you can get better over time. Fasting might feel a bit difficult and scary at first; you'll feel more hungry than usual, and the thought of not eating for hours or days at a time can be a hard mental block to get past. The more you fast, the stronger you'll get. The stronger you get, the easier fasting will become. This is exactly the same way that the more weights you lift and the bigger your muscles become, the stronger you'll get and the easier it will be to lift the weights.

So think about that the next time you're struggling—*you're building your fasting muscle*. Part of building your fasting muscle is realizing that feeling hungry and uncomfortable is a natural part of the journey, just like feeling muscle fatigue and burn is part of the journey at the gym. Every day, you're getting a little stronger, and every day it gets a little easier to fast. You might not see it and feel it immediately, but two weeks or a month from now, you'll look back and be amazed at how much stronger you've become. You get stronger only by pushing through and continuing to lift that figurative fasting barbell. If you give in, your fasting muscle will get weaker, and fasting will become much harder.

The fact is, we get better at doing the things we keep doing. So if you keep giving up every time you struggle, you're teaching yourself that giving in is the easiest option, and you're getting better at giving in. The same thing goes for staying strong. The more you stay strong and push through, the more you're teaching your body and your mind that that's the easier track—you're getting stronger at staying strong.

So when you're thinking about breaking, ask yourself if you want to be on the track where you're getting stronger and better at sticking to your goals, or do you want to be on the track where you're getting weaker and better at giving in? Do you want to train yourself to give up more, or do you want to train yourself to stay strong more?

To make the most consistent progress, you might want to start easy at first. You wouldn't lift the heaviest weights at the gym right away, and in the same way, you shouldn't throw yourself into a super long fast too early. Start with shorter fasts, and slowly extend them as you build your confidence and fasting muscle. Each time you push through challenging times, you're building both your mental and physical fasting strength.

Fasting isn't easy, and weight loss definitely isn't easy either. Some days it will be a breeze, and some days will be really tough. Having ups and downs like that is completely normal. What matters is how you're using your challenges to learn and grow and strengthen your fasting muscle. Just remember that you grow when you challenge yourself. If you cave and cut a fast short, it can slow down your progress, making it tougher to pick up speed again. Every day you're fasting—especially the hard days—helps you make your fasting muscle stronger and bigger.

COMBINING FASTING with EXERCISE

If you're worried about working out while fasting, don't be. Working out while fasting is not a problem, and fasting can actually improve your workouts.

Fasting can boost your human growth hormone (HGH) levels,[1] which is important for maintaining and growing your muscles and for your general physical health. So when your HGH levels are high, both your stamina and performance at the gym improve.

Many fitness enthusiasts and bodybuilders swear by fasted workouts because they know that fasting boosts fat-burning and keeps their energy steady without having a high-carb meal before a workout. When you work out in a fasted state, your body starts to burn more fat than it normally would for energy because there's no freshly consumed glucose to burn. And because fasted workouts lead to more fat-burning, they can give you better body composition in the long term. Another huge perk of fasted workouts is that they let you avoid the infamous "sugar crashes" that sometimes happen after you eat carbs and then exercise. On top of this, research has shown that eating a carb-heavy meal before your workout decreases fat-burning, whereas fasting for longer than six hours before a workout makes you burn more fat.[2]

As I've previously discussed, fasting puts your body through ketosis, where it shifts from using glucose from food for energy to using ketones from breaking down your fat. When you work out in a fasted state, you speed up this fat-breakdown process, and you have a virtually endless supply of energy to take from. The farthest I've ever run is a half marathon, and I did it in a fasted state. Running that far was completely unplanned, but I felt so good and full of energy that I had to keep going. My initial goal was to run a 5K, and I had been fasting for forty-eight hours already. On my run, I felt so energetic that I just kept on running until I'd completed a 10K, then a 15K, and then eventually a half marathon (13.1 miles). Because I was fasting, and I was already fat adapted, I was able to keep running with a steady supply of energy in a way that I'd never been able to do before I discovered fasting and keto. When you're used to eating a high-carb diet (as I was before), you experience sugar highs and crashes as your body burns through its stored glucose for energy. If you've ever watched a marathon on TV, long-distance runners usually have energy gels to boost their energy when they have a sugar crash. But because I was fat adapted and in a ketogenic state, I didn't need any crutches of that sort, and I didn't experience any sugar crashes or dips in energy even though it was such a long run.

Things to keep in mind when you're working out in a fasted state is to drink plenty of water and make sure to take an electrolyte supplement, especially during a long fast or a tough workout. Stay away from so-called electrolyte waters or electrolyte drinks, though. They don't give you enough of what you need and sometimes contain sweeteners and flavorings that will break your fast.

It's also important to listen to your body and ease yourself into working out in a fasted state. Start with easy exercises and increase the intensity as you get used to it. If you're feeling strong and full of energy, you can keep working out normally, but if you start to feel weak or dizzy, listen to your body and take a break or lower the intensity of your workout.

Finally, I want to emphasize that working out is *not* required to lose weight when you're fasting. The weight loss will come from the fasting itself and from switching to a ketogenic diet. Working out while fasting can be hugely beneficial, but only if it makes you feel good. If working out makes you feel stressed, there's no need to do it. Only work out if it makes you feel good and happy. Working out can be an excellent boost to your mood and to your physical and mental health, so make sure it feels like a boost and not a burden.

CLIENT SPOTLIGHT: TAMMY

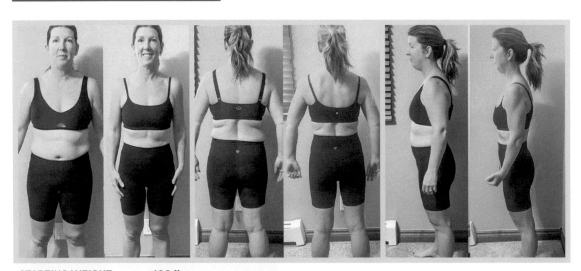

STARTING WEIGHT	160 lbs
CURRENT WEIGHT	125 lbs
TOTAL WEIGHT LOST	35.5 lbs

On January 1, 2024, I woke up and said, "I have to make a change and figure out how to reset my body and my choices and start feeling better physically and mentally." A friend had told me how fasting helped her meet her weight-loss goals, and she introduced me to a great coach to get me on the right track. I had seen all the ads for intermittent fasting but never thought it was for me or that it would be a long-term plan. However, I was wrong, and I am forever grateful that I gave intermittent and extended fasting a try. I started this journey for weight loss and have gained so much valuable information not only for weight loss but what it does to help heal your body.

I am 45 years old and had tried every fad diet that has come along. In the past, I've counted calories and increased my exercise but could never get the results that I was hoping to achieve. Over the years, the weight kept creeping on; I felt exhausted all the time and had aches in my knees, hips, and feet. I started to research weight-loss medication, but I knew that I wanted a lifestyle change that I could maintain, and I wanted to learn how to build a lifestyle that would continue to work for me.

When I first started the fasting journey, it wasn't easy, but I wanted change, so I followed the plan, started seeing results in the first few days, and continued to figure out the path that worked best for me. I started this journey at 160.5 pounds, and in the first twenty days, I started off with intermittent fasting and gradually worked up to extended fasting. I was excited with the weight loss; by Day 26, I was down 20 pounds, over 15 inches gone, and I was also feeling so much better! My aches were not noticeable, I was sleeping better, my unhealthy cravings had significantly improved, I started to see muscle definition, and my skin looked healthier than it had in years. This is exactly the reset I was hoping to find, and I have been able to discover a path that works for me. I have now achieved my goal weight of 125 pounds, and I feel better than ever. I still face challenges, but each challenge is a learning experience that helps me better understand how different foods and situations affect my body and health. Travel, stress, and eating out have all been hurdles for me, but fasting is a reset that has given me back the power to believe in myself and my body again.

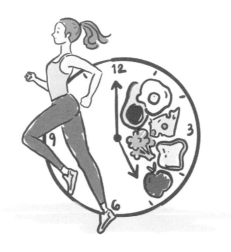

CHAPTER 9
GETTING OFF THE STRUGGLE BUS

When you're fasting, you're likely going to come across some difficult moments. For example, you might struggle with hunger, to balance your electrolytes, or with fitting fasting around your social schedule. In this chapter, I go over the most common fasting struggles and give you practical steps and tips to overcome them.

RECOGNIZING and OVERCOMING the SIDE EFFECTS of FASTING

Even if you're fasting correctly, it can have some undesirable physical side effects, especially if you're new to fasting or a ketogenic diet. The good news is that most of these unpleasant side effects will get better over time, and there are several things you can do to help minimize them or completely avoid them.

Keto Flu

When you're not used to fasting or a ketogenic diet, you can sometimes experience some unpleasant reactions as your body switches over to ketosis. You can feel weak, dizzy, nauseous, or tired—almost like you have the flu. This collection of side effects is known as *keto flu*, and it's the most common side effect of fasting or starting a ketogenic diet.

So why do you get keto flu? Most of the time, keto flu is a sign of carb withdrawal. Because you're most likely used to eating a standard Western or Standard American Diet, you're not used to burning body fat for fuel; you're used to burning food and carbs. In other words, your body is used to glycolysis, which is when your body breaks down outside sources of food, specifically carbohydrates, into energy. Moving away from glycolysis can temporarily make you feel some withdrawal symptoms.

Our ancestors regularly cycled through periods of fasting and feasting. The problem in modern society is that we're not used to the *fast* phase because we exist almost entirely in the *feast* phase. Every single day, seven days a week, 365 days a year, we're burning fuel from food and storing the rest. And because we're not tapping into the fast cycle regularly, we don't get to burn body fat; we just store it.

The reason you might feel some of these uncomfortable side effects when you switch to a ketogenic diet or start fasting is that your body needs to completely start up a system that has been inactive for years—maybe even your whole life. Starting a whole new system isn't easy, so you're going to experience some hiccups before it runs smoothly. Your body is so used to high-carb, high-sugar content in your diet that your body doesn't know how to cope when you suddenly deprive it of carbs. Fortunately, the symptoms of ketosis usually go away within two or three days as your body gets used to using this new system, especially as you become fat adapted.

Keto flu isn't dangerous, but it can be uncomfortable. So what can you do about it? The best way to decrease the symptoms of keto flu is to take electrolytes. You need sodium, potassium, and magnesium every single day when you're fasting or on a ketogenic diet to replace any minerals you lose through body fat and water weight.

Headaches, Weakness, or Tiredness

Other common side effects of fasting are headaches, weakness, and tiredness. Most of the time, these symptoms are a sign of low sodium levels. As soon as you start fasting, your insulin levels drop. Because insulin causes you to retain water, when your insulin levels drop, you release extra water, which is why you often have to pee a lot when you first start fasting or following a ketogenic diet.

When you flush out all that extra water, a lot of electrolytes go with it. Because you're not eating anything, you're also not replenishing the electrolytes through food.

Getting rid of headaches, weakness, and tiredness that result from fasting is usually as simple as taking some extra salt. You can sprinkle a little bit of pink salt or sea salt under your tongue, or you can add some to a glass of water. You can also try drinking some bone broth or taking a sip of unsweetened pickle juice. If your symptoms don't stop, you might have to consider breaking your fast.

Insomnia

When you start fasting, your body releases adrenaline, which is usually a good thing because it speeds up your metabolism and gives you more energy. But it's not so great at the end of the day when you want to go to sleep, and you may find that you experience some insomnia or feel like you have too much energy in the evening.

When you're fasting for the first time, it's common for you to toss and turn or feel like you've had too much coffee in the middle of the night. If you keep fasting, your body will get used to the increased levels of adrenaline, and the insomnia usually gets better.

Another thing to note is that you actually need less sleep when you're fasting. Because your body isn't spending any energy digesting food, you have a lot of energy left at the end of the day, meaning you need less sleep to recover. Your body is also still programmed to keep you awake so you can hunt for a big tasty animal, but as you know, that's not so relevant to you anymore.

Although fasting-related insomnia usually isn't dangerous, it can still be uncomfortable. To combat it, try turning off your electronics about an hour before bed or using blue light–blocking glasses in the evening. Both are good ways to help your brain switch off and get ready for bed. You can also try taking some extra magnesium a few hours before you go to bed because magnesium can help relax your muscles, increase melatonin, and decrease cortisol. If you find that you're unable to sleep despite your best efforts, it's better to get up and do something productive rather than tossing and turning. Try going to bed only when you're actually tired enough to fall asleep.

Acid Reflux

Some people get acid reflux when they first start fasting, but this side effect usually only affects those who have a history of reflux. It can be uncomfortable, but luckily there are some things you can do to make it better.

Taking a shot of apple cider vinegar in a glass of water a couple of times a day usually helps alleviate the symptoms. The reason is thought to be because apple cider vinegar is a probiotic that helps balance the good and bad bacteria in your gut. If you're having trouble with reflux, avoid drinking pickle juice, bone broth, and peppermint or spearmint teas because they can make the reflux worse.

Bad Breath

One of the most common side effects of fasting is bad breath. Bad breath while fasting is usually caused by ketosis; therefore, it's commonly known as *keto breath*. Keto breath happens because your body starts to break down your body fat for energy, and acetone is a by-product created from the process. When this happens, your tongue can turn white, you can have an acetone-like taste in your mouth, and your breath can smell sweet or like acetone. Some people describe keto breath as smelling like pear drops. Although it can be unpleasant, keto breath is a great sign that you're in ketosis and your body is burning fat for fuel, so definitely keep going.

Keto breath tends to settle as your body gets used to being in ketosis. In the meantime, brush your teeth as normal, and use a tongue scraper or brush your tongue throughout the day. Also make sure that you stay well hydrated because not drinking enough water can also cause bad breath. Avoid using mouthwash, though; the sweet taste of mouthwash could put you at risk for breaking your fast.

If you really want to be careful about not brushing your teeth with anything sweet during an extended fast, you can choose a natural toothpaste with no added sweeteners or flavorings. These toothpastes don't have any sugar or sweeteners, so they won't risk breaking your fast, and they clean your teeth just fine.

Balancing Your Electrolytes

To make sure you feel as good as possible and avoid side effects, you need to manage your electrolyte balance. You need sodium, potassium, and magnesium every single day when you're fasting, and it also helps to take electrolytes when you're on a ketogenic diet.

The easiest way to make sure you're getting the appropriate amounts of all these electrolytes is to take a complete electrolyte supplement every day. These come in pill, capsule, or powder form, and many people think that a pill or a capsule is easier to take than powder. If you use the powder form, you have to mix it with water, and the taste can be difficult to stomach.

When you're choosing an electrolyte supplement, be careful to read the back of the label. Most electrolyte supplements don't contain nearly enough of what you need every day, and many of them also contain sweeteners or flavorings that will break your fast. It's important that you know what you're getting.

In this section, I tell you how a deficiency of each electrolyte can affect you. If you experience any of these side effects, try increasing the corresponding electrolyte, and you should start to feel better.

LOW SODIUM

Signs of low sodium include headaches, nausea or vomiting, dizziness, brain fog, and general fatigue.

To fix it, try having a little bit of extra salt. You can place a pinch of sea salt or pink salt under your tongue and let it melt. The salt will go straight into your bloodstream quickly, which will even out any symptoms you're feeling that are due to low sodium.

LOW MAGNESIUM

The most common signs of low magnesium are muscle cramps or weakness, insomnia, irregular heartbeat, and irritability.

The best way to get extra magnesium while fasting is to take a magnesium supplement. Choose one that has approximately 500 mg of magnesium citrate, magnesium malate, or magnesium glycinate. Try to avoid using magnesium oxide because the body doesn't absorb it as well, and it can give you diarrhea.

LOW POTASSIUM

Low levels of potassium can result in stomach cramps, high blood pressure, a rapid heartbeat, constipation, numbness or tingling in your extremities, or a low mood.

To add extra potassium while you're fasting, mix ½ to 1½ teaspoons of potassium citrate powder with your water to get 1,000 to 3,000 mg of potassium. Alternatively, you could use 1 teaspoon of potassium chloride (available as NuSalt), which provides 3,180 mg of potassium.

Do NOT exceed daily maximum

Electrolytes	Symptoms	Total daily required Fasting/Keto Diet
Sodium	Headache Fatigue Nausea/vomiting Dizziness Brain fog	5,000 to 7,000 mg/day 1 teaspoon of salt = 2,335 mg sodium
Magnesium	Muscle cramps/weakness Irritability Insomnia Irregular heartbeat Headache/dizziness	300 to 500 mg/day Malate, glycinate, or citrate capsules or tablets
Potassium	Muscle cramps/weakness Nausea/vomiting Abdominal cramps High blood pressure Rapid heartbeat Constipation Numbness/tingling Depression	1,000 to 3,500 mg/day ½ to 1½ teaspoons potassium citrate powder provides 1,000 to 3,000 mg potassium 1 teaspoon potassium citrate (NuSalt) provides 3,180 mg potassium

CAUTION

Please note that so-called electrolyte waters or electrolyte drinks such as Gatorade are not fasting approved. They usually don't contain nearly enough of the electrolytes you need, many contain sweeteners, or both.

DEALING with HUNGER PANGS

Perhaps the most noticeable thing you're going to have to struggle with when you're fasting is hunger. A lot of us aren't used to dealing with hunger in any extensive way, so this can be quite a startling experience.

Hunger is an important biological and evolutionary response in your body. It's your body's way of protecting you and making sure you survive. Hunger signals you to start looking for food, and thousands of years ago, that meant getting ready to go on a hunt or a foraging trip. Now, you simply open the refrigerator door or drive five minutes to the closest supermarket.

From an evolutionary standpoint, the human body is still stuck in that old way of existing, even though society has developed at a quicker pace. So your brain is telling you, "Oh, my gosh, I need to go find food RIGHT NOW," as soon as you feel the slightest hunger pang, but if you give in to every last one of those, you'll eat way more than you need and gain weight. Your first challenge is realizing that hunger is normal and natural. It's a signal to start *thinking* about *maybe* looking for food at some point in the near future. You can view hunger as a suggestion rather than a command. And when you accept the reality that hunger is a part of fasting, the journey is going to be easier for you.

Next, you need to understand that hunger pangs are not dangerous. They're not going to do anything harmful to you, although they can be unpleasant. Nothing bad is going to happen if you ignore them.

The last piece is realizing that hunger comes and goes in waves. When you start to feel hungry, it doesn't get worse and worse without relief. If you wait it out, your hunger pang will reach a peak and then subside or even go away.

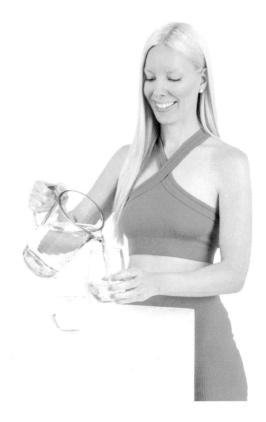

What's interesting is that we tend to feel hungry around breakfast time, lunchtime, and dinnertime because we've taught our bodies to expect food on that schedule. Hunger is something of a learned response. When you're constantly feeding your body food and snacks around the clock, you teach your body to *expect* food and snacks around the clock. Breaking that pattern is a crucial part in unlearning some of these excessive hunger cues.

Because hunger is uncomfortable but not dangerous, you can let your hunger sit with you. You don't have to act on it. Drink a glass of water, go for a walk, or distract yourself with an activity that you enjoy, and the hunger will soon go away.

If you can't shake the feeling of hunger, ask yourself if you're truly hungry. Are you actually just bored? Anxious? Sad? You eat for a variety of reasons, but many of them aren't because you're actually hungry. Tuning in to the true reasons behind *why* you're having cravings or thoughts about food is an important step to success on your weight-loss journey.

We're conditioned to panic when we feel hunger, but that panic isn't necessary. Most people have plenty of stored body fat to live on—for weeks. So when you're feeling hungry and it seems like the bells are ringing and the red lights are flashing, try to reframe that feeling into something *positive*. Say, "YES!" *Yes* to the changeover from burning sugar to burning fat. When you feel that hunger, you're fasting, and that's exactly what you wanted to do. When you feel that hunger, your body is tapping into your stored body fat for fuel, which is also what you wanted it to do. So instead of feeling panicked or scared of hunger, try instead to feel empowered by it. If you can get through an hour, you can get through a day, and you'll be building your fasting muscle every time you do.

FASTING THROUGH SOCIAL EVENTS

You'll have social events to attend while you're on a fasting or weight-loss journey. It's inevitable. After-work get-togethers, birthdays, weddings, and family dinners. You can't completely isolate yourself inside your home until you've reached your goal, so you need to have a clear strategy for how you'll deal with these situations.

Fasting can be difficult if you have a lot of social events because many occasions revolve around food in some way. I'm here to tell you that it *is* possible to do it as long as you do some mental preparation and planning.

One of the keys to fasting through food-oriented events or celebrations is to have scripted replies prepared. My favorite statements are along these lines:

- I'm not hungry.
- I already ate.
- I'm going to eat later.

Another alternative when someone offers you food is simply saying, "No, thanks." Remember, "No" is a complete sentence. You're a grown person, and no one can force you to eat anything that you don't want to eat.

It's easy to get caught up in the idea of "special occasions" or "celebrations" and that *other people* would be happy if *you* eat something. That's a risky mindset and a slippery slope. I grew up as a people pleaser, so this is something I've had to work on a lot. You're only responsible for yourself and your own happiness, and eating food is not a celebration for you right now. Instead, *not* eating food is a celebration. Your friends want you there to celebrate and spend time with them because they love you and want to have great conversations and hang out. You can still do those things without eating.

I've fasted through many events and family get-togethers. Here's one example: When my husband got a promotion, we planned a night out at a fancy Michelin-starred restaurant. On the date of the dinner, I was on a seven-day fast and couldn't partake in the food. But we still went together and enjoyed great conversation while he dined and I had a cup of peppermint tea. It was a lovely and special evening.

The first time I fasted at a family barbecue, I got some funny looks, but people got over it. And now, no one bats an eye.

I even fasted through my own wedding rehearsal dinner. Did people think I was weird? *You bet!* But I didn't care because I had more important things to focus on. After all those events, I walked away feeling amazing, strong, and accomplished.

Before you've done it for the first time, you can't really know what it'll feel like. You may be nervous about what other people will think, but stay focused on showing up for *your own* health and happiness, which starts by prioritizing yourself *every day.* No matter if there's a special occasion or not. You are a special occasion, no matter what other things are going on.

Anything is possible. You just have to make your mind up about what you want. If you don't, you'll easily find excuses not to fast. There will always be food-centered events and celebrations. But being there and celebrating with everyone is the most important thing. Not whether you're eating.

Focus on *your* journey. And realize that eating food is not the only way to celebrate. Celebrate by having meaningful conversations, laughing with the people you love, and spending time together.

DEALING with HATERS

When you commit to a lifestyle change, not everyone in your circle is going to be supportive. This is often because they have their own insecurities. The changes you're making are forcing them to take a good hard look at themselves, their behaviors, and the choices they may not be ready to confront.

Because of this, they might consciously or subconsciously make it harder for you to stick to your plan. They might try to make themselves feel better by actively sabotaging you by encouraging you to eat things you're trying to move away from. Or they might just forget that you're living your life differently now and offer you food that's not on your plan.

In these situations, you need to have a strong idea of your needs and boundaries. Remind yourself that every time you say "no," you recommit to your journey. When you're focused on your health and happiness, you sometimes need to set aside the feelings of the people around you. Compromising your own well-being doesn't help anyone in the long run—especially not you.

When people criticize or question your fasting, it can be helpful to have some responses prepared. Here are some examples:

- When people say, "Fasting is unhealthy; you should do this other diet instead, like me," try replying, "None of those things have worked for me. I'm trying this now, and I'd appreciate your support."

- When someone questions you, suggest that they research it. It's not your responsibility to educate anyone on fasting, and if people want more information, there are plenty of resources out there. A quick internet search will bring up a variety of information supporting the benefits of fasting, which will help to debunk any myths that fasting is bad for you.

- Saying that you're fasting for general health reasons can shift the conversation from focusing on weight to explaining that fasting is amazing for your overall health—physical, mental, and emotional—and it goes much further than just weight loss.

Try to be patient with the people around you and understand that your efforts to change can be challenging for them. Make sure you stay strong in your commitment to your goals, and don't let any haters get in your way.

PLATEAUS and STALLS

When you're fasting, you'll sometimes run into what is known as a stall or a plateau. After losing weight consistently for a while, your weight loss slows or comes to a complete stop even if you haven't changed anything in your daily routine.

It's generally not considered a stall until you've had two weeks of no weight loss at all. If your weight has been unchanged for only a few days, wait it out because the weight should start moving again soon.

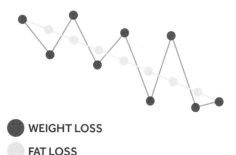

LOSING WEIGHT VS. LOSING FAT

Body weight will fluctuate weekly and even daily

● WEIGHT LOSS
○ FAT LOSS

Stalls and plateaus can be super frustrating, but they're usually nothing to worry about. In fact, the human body can fluctuate in weight by as much as 5 pounds in a single day. Weight goes up and down for many reasons, including what you've eaten the day before, how much you've had to drink, stress levels, or hormone levels—especially if you're a woman.

Troubleshoot your stall by thinking about whether you've done anything differently in the last few days that might explain this stall. Did you weigh at a different time? Did you eat or drink anything differently, or did you have a particularly high stress level at work? Are you due for your period? If none of those things are out of the ordinary, you can usually trust that your weight will get moving again in a couple of days.

In some cases when your weight loss stalls, you might be due for what's known as a *whoosh*. This is especially true when you've been losing weight consistently for a while, and then your weight suddenly shoots up, seemingly overnight, by a couple of pounds or more. This could be a sign that your body is getting ready to release some excess water weight. After a whoosh, you may lose 1 to 5 pounds of weight overnight.

Remember: Weight loss and fat loss are not necessarily the same thing, and weight loss doesn't happen in a straight line. It's normal for it to fluctuate slightly up and down weekly or even daily. As long as the overall trend is going down week by week, you know you're on the right track.

CLIENT SPOTLIGHT: FRANCES

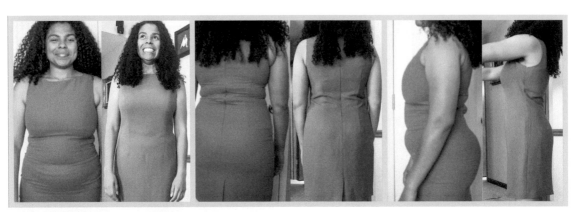

STARTING WEIGHT	162 lbs
CURRENT WEIGHT	132 lbs
TOTAL WEIGHT LOST	30 lbs

"Nothing tastes as good as skinny feels."

There are several things that may fuel a person's consistency. Mine was desperation. I felt disgusted and bloated. When I looked at photos of myself, I didn't recognize who I was.

Your weight does not define who you are. But it sure as hell makes you feel something you shouldn't.

I applaud the women who are comfortable in their skin at any weight. I almost envy them. Their mental health is stronger than mine will ever be.

But it wasn't just looks that fueled my motivation to lose weight; it was my allergies. The more inflammation that carbohydrates within my system created, the more I'd wheeze. The more I'd sneeze. The more sluggish I became. The more clogged my brain was.

When you fast, there comes a sense of clarity. Like a reset—a factory reset. And lawd knows, we need that on the daily.

Fasting changed my life. I lost 30 pounds, and it changed everything for me.

I was comfortable in my skin. I was comfortable in anything I wore. I was focused. I woke up before the sun came up. I accomplished tasks like I'd never done before.

It took some cranking to get the ol' fasting engine started, but once it did, I felt like I was on autopilot.

The best way to lose weight quickly, without constantly thinking about what you should and should not eat, the agonizing thought of "Ah, did I eat too much?" or questioning "Will this affect the scale at all?" is to fast.

I followed fasting plans for three months. The first month, I did alternate-day fasting (ADF). Sunday night at 7:00 p.m., I'd commence a forty-two-hour fast. I'd eat within a four-hour window on Tuesday afternoon and then fast another forty-two hours until Thursday. I'd next eat on Saturday and Sunday.

On days I feasted, my diet was strictly keto. Meat and veggies and occasionally some berries, heavy whipping cream, and cheese.

It was helpful to have a limit on what I could eat. It kept me focused without constant guesswork and preparation. "I've got a steak defrosted, broccoli I can steam, and a cheese snack—perfect. If I get hungry later on, I'll sip on some green tea. Emma says something warm always brings about a feeling of fullness."

During the second month, Emma introduced extended fasting to me. We started with fasting for seventy-two hours and increased each week, if my body and mind were able. The longest extended fast I was able to complete was ten days.

Once you have the ball rolling, you feel unstoppable. *Unstoppable.* Let me reiterate, the clarity that comes with fasting is unheard of. When I was fasting, I absolutely was On. My. Game. I was productive. I was moving. The best part of it all, I slept less. Without the need to digest three meals a day throughout the night, my body didn't require as much rest. I'd say that's a winner.

During my three months of fasting, I went from a whopping 161.8 pounds to 132.0. It was the fastest I've ever lost thirty pounds.

Three years have passed, and I still implement fasting in my day-to-day life. I remember that Emma explained how hunger comes in waves and how our relationship with food must change. She described how it should be viewed as a pleasure in moments of celebration and fuel on the other days. Every day is a celebration, but not every day should be celebrated with a feast.

Some of Emma's words still ring in my ear:

- "With fasting, let exercise become natural; exercise because you want to. Take a walk because you want to."
- "Our bodies don't need extra fuel when exercising. It already has plenty stored up—those fat storages!"
- "You've got to eat for the body you are aiming for, and naturally, it'll get there."

The crucial part is to look at fasting as more than just a habit you practice for a few months and then abandon. Your body becomes accustomed to that minimal food intake; you've got to learn to listen to it.

Like with anything that's a wee bit tough in life, if it's easy, everyone would be doing it.

SUSTAINING FASTING LONG TERM

To be successful in the long run, you need to accept that fasting isn't just a diet. It's a lifestyle change for the long haul because it isn't just about losing weight.

You can reap all the other health benefits that come along with it. So even after reaching your weight goal, you can use fasting for health benefits like autophagy, reducing inflammation, and improving your mood.

What does successful long-term fasting look like?

You need to find a fasting schedule that works for you long term. For example, even in maintenance, I usually fast at least sixteen hours every single day. It's a schedule that works well for me and my lifestyle.

The beauty of fasting is that it's flexible. You can tailor it to fit with your work and social life. If you frequently have lunch meetings at work, adapt your eating windows so it fits around that obligation. If you have family dinner every night, your fasting window can easily be tailored around that. The 16:8 schedule is usually an easy and manageable routine for most people to fit into their lifestyles.

For long-term fasting success, don't view trips, celebrations, and special events as hindrances. Instead, plan so that you can fit these social occasions into your life as comfortably and seamlessly as possible.

Remember that fasting for weight loss is a journey. As with any journey, there will be ups and downs. Make sure that you take each moment, good or bad, as a learning opportunity, reminding yourself that it's not about the number of times you fall down but the number of times you get back up and move forward that counts.

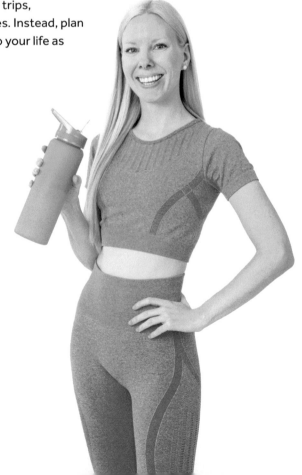

CLIENT SPOTLIGHT: MANDY

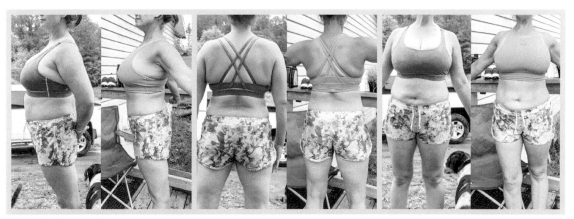

STARTING WEIGHT	**160.7 lbs**
CURRENT WEIGHT	**143.4 lbs**
TOTAL WEIGHT LOST	**17.3 lbs**

Fasting! It's life-changing. It's phenomenally healthy! It's transformative! And without a doubt, it's the best thing I've ever done for myself and my body! BOOM! But there are some damn deep lows too; this isn't an easy change to start or stick with.

I've *always* wanted to be thinner: always. I've learned over the last few years that I actually was never that heavy to begin with. But now that I'm over 40, I have a lot more challenges to contend with. I became heavier than ever before, and I put on weight in the blink of an eye.

I *never* lost weight through exercising. I was mowing lawns with a push mower and serving at a restaurant at night. I could easily have more than 45,000 steps in one day, and I frequently walked 12 miles (20 km) in a day. To me, this was both a phenomenal accomplishment and a totally frustrating and disappointing learning experience. I was astounded that I could do so much physical activity, but I couldn't lose a single pound!

I *cannot* lose weight unless I do some serious fasting. Fasting just *makes sense*. It makes sense for losing weight, and it makes sense for maintaining weight. There's absolutely no reasoning behind the idea that we should eat more to lose weight. It's completely counterintuitive, and if you're diabetic, eating more makes the disease worse.

I started fasting slowly. To begin, I stopped eating breakfast. Then I quit taking a lunch to work and dropped the carbs. During the busy summer, I wouldn't eat until I was done working both jobs at 10:00 p.m., and I always ate keto. This was amazing for my body, and I felt great.

I discovered I can eat one meal a day and maintain my weight. To lose weight, I need to eat supper every second day. That is what works best for me. Is it easy? Absolutely not, but I'm teaching myself not to binge and not get that desperate feeling like I'm never going to eat again. I've had some extremely bad habits over the years, and if there's one thread that runs through them all, it's bingeing. Food is all I have left, and it's taking some determination to remove that desperate, stuff-my-face feeling from the equation. But I *am* doing it.

With fasting, I lost 17 pounds in thirty days. I went from 160.7 pounds to 143.4 pounds.

I'll never stop fasting. I'll never go back to eating more than twice a day, and eating twice is only a once-a-week thing. When I do eat more than once a day, it's too much food, and I don't enjoy my supper because I'm still full from breakfast or brunch.

Frequent extended fasts are still difficult for me to manage. I have to learn how to not let the refeed throw me into a binge session, and I have a lot of work to do to maintain myself mentally through a longer fast. Physically, I'm fine, and I'm not hungry a bit. But it's hard to stay rational each day, and I find myself obsessing about food. But don't get me wrong: I *can* and *will* do longer fasts.

It's all brain work, and I have a brain, so I can do it. A ten-day fast is my big goal. Eating is my happy time, as I think it is for a lot of people. Fasting is a tool to allow us to manage our eating habits and weight without drugs and without damaging our metabolism. If you try fasting, you'll never feel better! And the health benefits are amazing—fasting improves your longevity, autophagy, gut health, and brain health. There is simply nothing else you can do for your body that can benefit your life more!

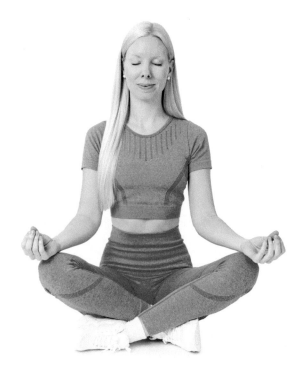

CHAPTER 10
GETTING YOUR MINDSET RIGHT

I want to tell you something: You're not broken. I used to think I was broken. I used to think just because I had a hard time losing weight there was something physically wrong with me. I thought perhaps I had a problem with my thyroid, or I was genetically predisposed to weight gain. I was so convinced that there was something physically wrong that was getting in my way that I sent off strands of my hair to be analyzed for a food intolerance that made it impossible for me to lose weight. When it came back, I was sorely disappointed. There was nothing wrong with me, and there's nothing wrong with you.

There's nothing unusual about you that's making it impossible for you to lose weight. Your starting point is identical to millions of other people. You may have some hormonal imbalances and mindset issues to work on, but at the core, you're normal, and you're not broken. And the sooner you can come to terms with that, the sooner you can start working and get to your goals.

Weight loss requires two things: commitment and consistency. So far, you've been lacking consistency. Although you feel like you've tried everything, the reason nothing has worked is that you haven't stayed with it long enough. You stay with a new schedule for two weeks, and then you say it's not working, so you go back to eating a highly processed, high-carb, high-sugar diet, and you gain even more weight. Then you tell yourself the diet isn't working. But in reality, *you're* not working. The fact is, you're not putting in the work to get the results, and *that's* the problem. If you're serious about losing weight, you need to commit and stay consistent. The weight you want to lose took years to gain, so it's not going to take only two weeks to lose. You need to stay with it longer for it to work.

In this chapter, I share techniques you can use to get your mindset right to stick with fasting for the long haul.

BUILDING a POSITIVE MINDSET

Fasting is a great way to commit to becoming healthier, but commitment isn't enough. How you approach your journey and the mindset you have will make a huge difference in your results. For your best chance at success, you need to build a positive, calm, and centered mindset, and you should never approach fasting from a stressed or punishing place.

Be as Positive as Possible

Never approach fasting from a negative or punishing mindset. If you cast fasting in a negative light, it will feel daunting, and it almost becomes a chore—something you have to get through even though you don't really want to. This mindset not only takes the joy out of your weight-loss journey but also can really hinder your progress.

You should always approach fasting with a positive mindset, and you should see it as an opportunity to grow and improve both physically and mentally. Make sure you approach each fast with lots of positive energy and excitement. When you're in a positive mindset, you'll be able to push yourself so much further, and you won't be tempted to give up nearly as much as when you approach fasting from a negative mindset.

Have a Calm, Centered Mindset

You also need to reduce your stress levels and approach fasting from a calm and centered space. Stress is one of the biggest triggers for emotional eating, and it makes fasting a lot more challenging. Because of this, you need to put habits in place that help with your emotional well-being. Calming activities help you manage your stress, reduce your anxiety, and keep you focused on your fasting goals while staying centered.

Try to think of activities that actively make you feel calmer. Examples include going for a walk, meditating, talking to a friend, or doing breathing exercises. Practice calming activities that work for you every day to actively stay on top of your mental and emotional well-being and keep your stress levels low.

One of the best ways to center yourself is to use a technique called grounding. To practice grounding, you lie down on the ground or the floor. The location is important; don't lie down on a couch or bed. You need to be directly on the ground (or on concrete or ceramic tile floor if you're indoors) to increase your skin-to-earth contact. Having contact with the ground helps electrical currents from the earth conduct through your body. Grounding has been shown to have positive effects on stress levels and general well-being,[1] so starting your day with a grounding exercise or using grounding when you're feeling your stress levels rising is an excellent tool to have in your fasting toolbox.

Be Kind to Yourself

Part of being positive is being kind to yourself. It's impossible to be "perfect" all the time. There will be days where you feel powerful, prepared, and successful, and there will be days where you're feeling down and like nothing is going your way. No matter what happens, always treat yourself with kindness every step of the way, and remind yourself that each step, no matter how challenging or small it is, is a step in the right direction. Every time you have a misstep, you learn something about yourself, so take the time to reflect, journal, and plan ways to avoid similar situations in the future. Having self-compassion builds your strength and positivity, which will make fasting so much more enjoyable and effective.

Focus on Fasting as Self-Care

Try to see fasting as an act of self-care rather than deprivation, punishment, or restriction. When you're fasting, you're *choosing* a healthier lifestyle, and you're *choosing* to give your body a break from highly processed foods and constant overeating; you're allowing your body to heal and detoxify. Shifting your perspective in this way changes the focus from what you're *losing* (your favorite processed foods, eating around the clock) to what you're *gaining* (health, weight loss, mental clarity). Shifting your frame of mind reminds you that fasting is the most loving thing you can do for yourself, and this gives you more encouragement to keep a positive mindset.

FINDING MOTIVATION

One of the most common issues to deal with when you start a new health or fitness journey is staying motivated. Many people think that to achieve your goals of losing weight, eating healthier, or going to the gym, you need to be motivated to do so. And if you're not motivated, it's going to be much harder for you to get there.

However, long-term success lies in turning the concept of motivation on its head. Motivation isn't something that's just going to come to you. You're not going to suddenly "find motivation." No one else can give you motivation because motivation can't come from outside influences. You're not going to wake up one day and suddenly be motivated to lose all your excess weight and then be able to keep that motivation high enough for long enough to reach your goals. Motivation is quite fickle. You can be completely motivated to start your diet on Sunday night, but come Monday evening, you've forgotten all about that motivation, and you're knee-deep in a tub of ice cream.

So forget about motivation, and *just do it*. The key is to understand that *action feeds motivation*. When you're doing something and making decisions that push you further along the path to achieving your goals, you're going to feel motivated to keep doing those things. Do the action first, and the motivation will follow.

You often trip yourself up by thinking too much about how you *should* do it, whether you'll be *able* to do it, how *long* it'll take you to do it, and how to stay *motivated*, but all of that head chatter is just holding you back from actually *doing it*. So don't worry about motivation; turn off your brain and just do what you need to do. When you do that, you'll soon be filled with so much inspiration, energy, and motivation just from *performing* the actions that reaching your goals will become much easier.

GOAL SETTING and VISUALIZATION

The physical aspect of weight loss is only one part of fasting. The mental and emotional part of the equation is just as important—if not more important—to reaching your goals. One of the most powerful sayings is, "Whether you believe you *can*, or whether you believe you *can't*, you are right."

So many people start a fast while saying, "I'll try my best," or "I hope I can make it to the end of this fast." But when you make statements like that, you've already failed because you don't even believe in your own ability to succeed at the goal that you've set yourself. Those types of statements mean you're starting from a place of doubt and disbelief in your own abilities to succeed and follow through. The key to success is changing doubt into genuine belief.

Believe in Yourself

What you believe about yourself shapes your physical reality. Fasting with a belief and conviction that you will achieve your weight-loss goals helps you make sure that you succeed at doing just that.

The same goes for *not* believing in yourself. When you're convinced that you can't do it or it's not working, then guess what happens. It won't.

This concept that belief shapes reality is not just philosophical; it's rooted in psychological research. Studies have shown that having positive expectations and beliefs about your ability affect how well you perform in sports and even how well you recover from surgery.[2]

The easiest way to demonstrate the power of belief is by examining the placebo effect. Studies on the placebo effect have shown that simply *believing* that a medicine will work is enough to make it work. This means that patients who are given sugar pills instead of the real medicine will sometimes experience the effects associated with the real medicine even when they haven't taken it.[3] This proves that the power of belief and the power of the mind are not intangible or imaginary but have real-life effects on your body and the physical world.

And you can apply the same principle to fasting. When you believe that you can succeed, you increase your motivation, strength, and ultimately your ability to succeed at what you set out to do. The key to success in fasting, and in any other life challenge for that matter, is convincing yourself of your absolute ability to achieve your goals, which in turn will activate a positive feedback loop that brings you forward and closer to your goals.

Because if you don't believe it, you'll never achieve it. But when you believe in your capacity to overcome challenges and reach your goals, you're more likely to engage in behaviors that align with those beliefs, such as sticking to your fasting schedule and making healthier food choices. And of course when you engage in those behaviors, it will translate into actual success.

Visualize Your Success

Visualization goes hand in hand with belief. *Visualization* simply means imagining as clearly as you can the desired outcome you have for yourself in the future. Visualization is more than wishful thinking. It's a powerful tool for priming your brain for success.

In the case of weight loss, visualization is imagining yourself in your thinner body or at your goal weight. It goes beyond what you look like. Visualization means completely stepping into that future version of yourself and imagining how your life will be affected overall. What does your new body feel like? What are you thinking about? What activities are you doing? How do you talk, walk, and act when you're in that new body? By vividly imagining yourself achieving your fasting and weight-loss goals, you engage the pathways in your brain in a way that mirrors the actual experience of achieving those goals. You're basically tricking your brain into thinking you're already there, which means that living in a way that will allow you to physically get there is much easier.

Research has shown that the brain can't really tell the difference between real and imagined scenarios. Both stimulate similar neural pathways within the brain. In fact, visualization activates the same neural pathways involved in actual behavior. One study, which looked at the effects of positive visualization on strength training, found that athletes who positively visualized themselves performing heavy lifts saw a 10- to 15-pound increase in the amount of weight they were able to lift, compared to their baseline performance.[4] Another study found that simply visualizing strongly using a specific muscle group was enough to increase the strength of that muscle by up to 53 percent.[5]

This is also why imagining a situation can create a strong emotional response within you. For example, if you imagine that you failed a test or a performance review at work, it'll make you feel horrible, and it will make you *feel* like you actually failed. Because your brain thinks that the imagined situation is real to a certain extent, it triggers an emotional response to the situation. But this also means that through visualization, you can "practice" success by imagining positive outcomes, which makes you more prepared for those situations and more likely to engage in actions that will make your goals happen.

This is also why avoiding negative visualization is so important. Regardless of whether you visualize a positive or negative outcome, the physical world will align with what you imagine. So, if you visualize yourself never achieving your goals, not being strong enough, or always giving up, then guess what. That's going to become your reality. It takes the same amount of effort to imagine a negative outcome as it takes to imagine a positive outcome, and neither outcome has happened yet. So why not visualize a positive outcome? It doesn't matter so much whether you believe in the visualized outcome yet. Think of it as a "fake it 'til you make it" scenario: The more you visualize and believe in something, the more you're going to take that on board, and the more those beliefs and visualizations are going to become your reality.

By regularly visualizing your goals and your success, you are essentially training your brain and body to perform the actions necessary to achieve them. Because in your mind, you've already succeeded.

To help you practice visualization, the next few sections suggest some exercises you can try.

EXERCISE 1

Start by writing down your goals. Make sure you include as much detail as possible, such as the number of hours you want to fast each day, how much weight you want to lose, how many glasses of water you want to drink, or how long you want to walk each day. Also write down why these goals are important to you.

Then create a vision board to give you a visual representation of where you want yourself to be. Your vision board can be on paper or on your laptop or phone. The main goal is to collect pictures and quotes that represent your goals and where you see yourself in the future.

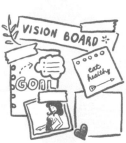

Then spend a few minutes every day looking at your vision board, imagining yourself in that space, and thinking about your goals. When you do this every day, you make sure that your focus is always on being in a positive and successful place rather than thinking about things you are unhappy with.

EXERCISE 2

Find a quiet and comfortable space where you can be by yourself for five minutes without anyone interrupting you. This can be your bedroom, your office, or, if you don't have a lot of space, even locked in the bathroom for a few minutes. As long as you're by yourself, any space is fine.

Once you're in your space, close your eyes and take time to truly visualize yourself achieving your fasting and weight-loss goals. Visualize yourself achieving your goal weight, loving your body, and making healthier food choices. Whatever your goals mean to you, vividly visualize them, as if you're already there. You should also visualize yourself overcoming every struggle you face. Imagine yourself easily pushing through every hunger pang or going for a walk instead of giving in and having a snack. When you vividly visualize, you're practicing making those things happen in reality.

For a visualization to be as successful as it can be, use all your senses to make it as vivid as possible. Think about what you see, hear, feel, and even smell when you've achieved your goal. The more real you can make the scenario in your head, the more successful the visualization exercise will be.

Finally, focus on the positive emotions that achieving your goal will give you. You may feel happy, feel satisfied in your body, love your new clothes, or be proud of yourself. The more you live in these feelings, the more real they're going to become, and the more likely you are to achieve your goals.

EXERCISE 3

Once you've practiced thinking about the ideal future version of yourself and you have a really clear picture of what that looks like, you need to start practicing "living as if." This means that you completely step into the person you want to become. Let go of any previous versions or ideas you have of yourself and start living like the person you want to be. For this to be successful, you need to identify as and act like that person completely.

Make a list of all the things your ideal self does each day. What does your morning routine look like? What do you have (or not have) for breakfast? How do you dress, eat, and talk about yourself? Do you work out?

Whatever your concept of your ideal self is, start to actively live like that right now. You might not be at your goal weight yet, but when you start living as if you already are, you'll achieve your goal weight much quicker.

Overcome Self-Sabotage and Negative Self-Talk

When you're on this fasting journey, you'll have good days and bad days. You may follow the plan perfectly for a few days, and then the next day, you might find yourself giving in to one of your excuses. That's just reality, and you need to be prepared for those ups and downs. But even if you've had a slipup or didn't quite make it to your fasting goal for the day or week, don't beat yourself up.

Don't dwell on the situation and make yourself feel bad about it. The key is not to let any negative emotions come in and destroy all the hard work you've put in. Instead, make sure you surround yourself with positivity and good thoughts. If you want to break your bad habits, you have to stay positive, especially when you're an emotional or anxious eater.

The reason this is so important is that when you make yourself feel bad about a decision you made, you create anxiety. And when you're feeling anxious, you're going to struggle to stay on plan, and you're more likely to self-sabotage. So you're just shooting yourself in the foot if you give those negative thoughts and feelings any room. When you have a positive mindset instead, you'll feel less stressed, anxious, and sad, so you'll be less likely to give in to bad habits and more empowered to push through and choose the right thing.

You can't hate yourself into having a body you love. Think about that for a second. You need to make sure that you love yourself through this whole journey, in good times and in bad. When you're struggling, take a deep breath and remind yourself that progress isn't linear and you're learning every step of the way. As long as you keep learning and keep trying, you're doing great!

Fix Your Default Thinking

To prevent yourself from going out of control after you've had a slipup, you need to change your default thinking, which is the immediate knee-jerk thoughts your brain presents as the truth in response to a given situation. Let me give you an example.

Think about a typical day: You start out great, with all your meals planned and your fasting window locked in. You have your keto lunch, drink plenty of water, and even do great at dinner. Then, when evening comes, you get impulsive thoughts to open the cupboard. You give in and have a snack. This is where your default thinking kicks in. You may have thoughts like these:

- "Screw it. I've ruined everything. I might as well throw it all out the window, go on a binge, and start over again tomorrow."
- "I'm a failure."
- "I don't even know why I bother anymore."

Next thing you know, you've scarfed down half the contents of the fridge, freezer, and cupboards, and you're left feeling guilty and deflated.

This chain of thoughts is your default thinking. But those thoughts aren't the truth. When you choose to believe these thoughts, you feel a lot of shame and regret. And your default thinking affects the choices you make in the wake of these thoughts. So you get trapped in a negative spiral of bad decisions made worse by these negative, and untrue, thoughts.

To break this pattern, you need to recognize your default thinking and change it to something better before it causes a chain reaction of unfavorable decisions. One slip on your fasting journey doesn't mean that your entire journey is messed up. The significance you give to slips seriously affects how well you're going to be able to move forward from them. The key is to try to alter your default thinking. When you trap yourself into the all-or-nothing mindset, you think, "I failed, so I might as well quit completely." But this way of thinking is holding you back, so you need to train your brain to switch to a more positive default thinking pattern.

The first step in changing your default thinking is recognizing that default thinking is happening in the first place. Because if you don't recognize that the default thinking is happening, you're going to keep making decisions based on it, which is going to cause you to eat more and self-sabotage more. The second step is separating what you *did* from what it means. One slip doesn't mean you're a failure and you've ruined everything. It simply means that you had one slip. So don't make the situation bigger than it has to be. Instead of thinking, "Eff it, I've messed up, so I might as well throw everything out the window and start again tomorrow," think, "OK, I messed up. No biggie. Let me learn from it and move on."

Your default thinking isn't set in stone; it's a habit that you built over time, which means you can change this type of thinking by being aware of it, catching it before it spirals you out of control, and working on switching it around. When you choose to change your default thinking, you'll find it so much easier to make choices that align with your goals.

PUSHING THROUGH HARD TIMES

You also need to be able to push through hard times when you're tempted to quit or cheat on your weight-loss journey. It's unrealistic to think you'll never experience struggles, and if you don't prepare for how you're going to react during those times, you're preparing yourself to fail.

In this section, I suggest some ways you can set yourself up to handle the challenging times.

Choose Your Track

Every time the voices of doubt come into your mind, or when the hunger and cravings seem completely unbearable, you need to stop and think carefully about your next steps. Because what you do in the next moments will have a massive impact on your ability to succeed on your weight-loss journey overall.

You need to ask yourself whether you're going to give in or push through and finish what you committed to. Pushing through a difficult time will fill you with a feeling of success and make you stronger. On the other hand, if you give in, you'll be left feeling awful, which will make you weaker. You probably already know that these scenarios are true because you've probably been through them before. So make sure you imagine what choosing the positive track will result in and what choosing the negative track will result in.

The bottom line is that positive actions create positive momentum, and negative actions create negative momentum. So every time you're tempted to quit or give in, you have to ask yourself whether you want to be on the positive track or the negative track.

Choosing to give in to a craving isn't limited to that one isolated decision. What you choose to do will impact all of your future decisions—and no, I'm not exaggerating. You're always progressing, but the question is, what are you progressing toward? You're either making decisions that push you toward success, reaching your goals, and feeling good about yourself, or you're making decisions that push you toward failure, being back where you started, and feeling bad about yourself. You are completely in control of which track you choose.

Build Trust in Yourself

The number one reason you're struggling with your weight is because you're a liar. Now, that might sound harsh, but hear me out.

Every time you've started a new diet, you've never followed through. And the same probably goes for a number of fasts you've started but not followed through on. When you do that enough times, you're teaching yourself that giving up is what you do best.

You might not think it's that big of a deal, but by breaking these small promises you've made to yourself, you're teaching yourself that you're not a trustworthy person. You're teaching yourself that when you make promises or commitments to yourself, you don't follow through on them. And that sets a dangerous precedent.

If you make a promise to your friends or your family, you follow through, right? If you didn't, people would start to think you're unreliable, and they wouldn't like you very much. So why aren't you treating yourself with as much respect?

The reason you don't keep those promises to yourself is because you're comfortable with failing, and you've started to identify yourself as being the type of person who fails. Being in this mindset is completely detrimental to your weight-loss success.

You need to start teaching yourself that you're the kind of person who *follows through* and sticks to promises you've made to yourself. The first step in doing that is never to commit to a fasting plan you're not realistically sure you can actually do. Once you've committed to a fasting plan, you complete it. *No excuses*. When you do that, you'll slowly start rebuilding your trust in yourself and start to see yourself as the kind of person who keeps their word.

When you build a strong foundation of trust in yourself, it's much easier to push through the hard times.

Parent Yourself

A great strategy to push through the hard times is to parent yourself. You've probably given in to cravings a hundred times before or said you would start a diet tomorrow but haven't followed through. A highly effective way to get out of that damaging spiral is to pretend you're your own parent.

Picture yourself as a child. Start viewing your defiant self—the one who doesn't follow rules and who just wants to eat cookies and ice cream all the time—as your "inner child." View your sensible self—the one who wants to lose weight, get healthier, and stick to their goals—as your "parent self." Separating those two personas will make your journey much easier and allow you to reach your goal weight with much less effort. It creates a psychological distinction between a smaller and weaker part of you (your child self) and a larger and stronger part of you (your parent self), which helps you overpower your negative thinking patterns.

When you start to parent your inner child, how you relate to everything you do in life will change—whether it's weight loss, work deadlines, health goals, or anything else you want to do that requires some effort and discipline—because it completely stops the negotiation.

My mom was an expert at this. If you grew up with a firm parent, you know that when they told you to do something (or not do something), you did as you were told. There was no negotiation. "Can I have three ice creams?" No. "Can I stay out late with my friends?" No. "Can I have birthday cake for breakfast?" The answer was no. It was a straightforward no, and even if you tried to argue, it didn't work. Negotiation was fruitless because your parent already decided that it was a no.

If you want to be successful on this weight-loss journey, you need to start treating yourself in the same way. When you have committed to a goal, there are just some things that are nonnegotiable. You decide what those are, but once they're decided, use your inner parent to make sure you stick to them. "Can I break my fast early?" No. "Can I have pizza because my friend is visiting?" No. "Can I bend the rules just a little bit?" No.

Parenting yourself is a great technique because it saves you from all the mind chatter and the back-and-forth negotiation. It's just no. Once you get into that mindset and you learn how to parent your inner child, you'll find pushing through hard times so much easier.

Keep Your Focus on the Right Things

Earlier in the chapter, I discussed how the way you talk to yourself plays a huge role in your success at achieving your goals. More than that, your thinking, and what you choose to focus on, has a huge impact.

When you focus on negatives, such as how unhappy you are with your weight and the idea that you've never been able to succeed on a weight-loss journey before, you take yourself further away from achieving your goals. This is because of the law of attraction, which says that the thoughts, feelings, and energy you put out in the world is what you're going to get back. So if you focus on all the things you *don't* want—you don't want to be this weight, you hate your body, you feel horrible—that's the energy you're putting out there, and that's what you're going to get more of.

If you instead focus on what you *do* want—feeling good, loving your body, being happy and healthy—you'll get more of that in return. If your mind is preoccupied with the things that you want to cut out of your life, you're actually pulling those things toward you instead. On the other hand, if you shift your focus to the things you're striving for, you'll invite more of those things into your life.

MAKE AFFIRMATIONS WORK FOR YOU

Affirmations are short, positive statements you repeat to yourself to help you overcome challenges and change your mindset. If you're trying to have a more positive mindset about work, you may tell yourself, "I love my job," or "I'm most productive and happy when I'm at work."

Positive affirmations are scientifically proven. Using affirmations to imagine positive events has been found to trigger the same areas in your brain that would be activated if the events happened in real life.[6]

For positive affirmations to be effective, they need to be specific, personal, and based in emotion, and they need to be in the present tense. Here are some weight-loss-oriented examples:

- "Fasting is easy for me."
- "I lose weight effortlessly."
- "I love eating unprocessed food."

When you use affirmations, you claim a future reality as if it's currently happening, which is why they need to be in the present tense.

Avoid using negative language in your affirmations. Instead of saying, "I don't want to struggle with cravings," try "I am in control of my hunger, and I make healthy food decisions easily."

Start your day by repeating your affirmations loudly to yourself several times. Doing so helps you rewire your brain to make those statements true.

GET OUT OF THE FOOD SCARCITY MINDSET

One of people's biggest fears when they start a fasting journey is that they will feel uncontrollably hungry. A lot of people try to avoid that situation by overeating during their mealtimes so they'll feel less hungry later. This way of thinking is completely wrong and one of the biggest things I work on with my clients to understand. Thinking that eating more during your eating window will make you feel less hungry during your fasting window is not true.

In fact, eating until you're stuffed won't delay hunger by much at all. Hunger and fullness are hormonal responses, and they aren't solely driven by the amount of food in your body. This is why you can feel full even when you're on the third day of an extended fast or why morbidly obese people can feel uncontrollably hungry despite eating copious amounts of food around the clock. Eating until you're stuffed at every meal out of fear of hunger is not a sustainable way to live. It's counterproductive because it will stop you from losing weight.

The underlying problem is your fear of hunger, so it's important for you to release that fear. The best way to think about hunger is that it isn't dangerous, and it's not going to harm you. Hunger is a natural response, and although it can be uncomfortable, it's usually nothing to worry about. A lot of us have learned hunger responses due to eating a lot, and many people also confuse cravings (mental hunger) for physical hunger. Cravings and hunger are not the same, and it's OK to have a craving without immediately doing something about it. It's also OK to have physical hunger without doing anything about it. Learn to be comfortable with hunger, and learn to separate actual hunger from cravings.

Try to reframe your view of hunger as something positive and something to welcome rather than fear. Feeling hungry means that you're fasting—which is what you want to do. Feeling hungry also means you're using your stored body fat for energy rather than food—which is also what you want. So anytime you feel that hunger coming on, don't be scared and panic. Instead, see it as something positive and a signal that you're doing all the right things for your weight-loss journey.

The other thing you need to deal with is your food-scarcity mindset. This is when you feel like you have to finish all the food *right now* because you're not sure of when you're going to be able to have this food again in the future. I've been there many times myself, finishing a whole box of doughnuts or several pints of ice cream in one sitting because "the diet starts tomorrow." Giving in to this way of thinking only increases your risk for overeating or binge eating (see the doughnut and ice cream example), and it makes you struggle even more to lose weight. It's also flawed thinking because food isn't going anywhere. The food you want right now is still going to be there when your fast is over or when you decide that it's an appropriate time for you to have that food.

Focus on the Action, Not the Result

It can be really tempting to focus on the finish line—losing 50 or 100 pounds (or however much weight you need to lose to fit in your clothes or look good at a specific event). Unfortunately, you can get so hung up on the result, on reaching your goal weight, and on how long it's going to take you to get there that you accidentally block yourself from achieving it. You build it up so much in your head that the goal can seem too far away or too hard to reach, especially if you aren't seeing progress as quickly as you want to. Sustainable weight loss isn't just about the goal. It's about how you get there.

To be successful in fasting for weight loss, you need to focus on the action, not the result. Instead of focusing on the huge end goal, how much weight you need to lose by next week, or how long it'll take you to get to your goal, try to focus on the small actions required of you every day: sticking to a keto diet, maintaining your fasting schedule, drinking water, and keeping a calm and positive mindset. When you place your focus on the smaller things, you're less preoccupied with all the stuff you can't control right now (such as exactly how much weight you'll lose by Friday or exactly how long it'll take you to reach your goal weight). Your mind is busy with the stuff you actually *can* control, such as drinking eight glasses of water a day or pushing through a hunger pang. When you focus on performing the actions that are required of you every day, you'll achieve your goals before you know it.

Focus on the action, not the result, and the results will follow.

Stop Being a Victim

A really important step in creating success for yourself is to get rid of the victim mindset. You need to stop blaming outside events for your actions or inactions and start seeing yourself as being in charge and owning your life choices.

You need to remember that there are no accidents. I often hear clients say, "I accidentally broke my fast," or "I accidentally ate a piece of candy." Of course, those statements are just BS. There are no accidents when it comes to this. Everything that happens and doesn't happen is a result of actions that you *choose* to take.

I know it can be really tempting to say that you *had* to eat because your relatives were in town or that you *had* to have dessert because otherwise your friends would think you're weird, but that is just a cop-out. You need to accept that. It was *your* choice to break your fast, your choice to eat the dessert, and your choice to eat because your friends or relatives were in town. That doesn't mean those choices were bad or that you're never allowed to eat or change your plans. You certainly can. It only means you need to realize that *you* are in control—no one else. Brutal accountability is key.

Owning your actions is the first step. When you have a victim mentality, you try to pass off control and decision-making to somebody else, and you look at yourself as some innocent creature who unfortunate things just happen to. But you always have a choice. You are a grown person, and you make your own decisions. What your mom, your auntie, and your friends think of your fasting is none of your business. You have to take ownership of what you do and empower yourself to take decisions. You are in control of your life. Until you recognize and own that, you will never be successful.

So it's important to change how you think about your actions. When you're at a party and there's a huge, delicious-looking cake there, you might think, "I can't eat that because I'm not allowed to." But thinking this way keeps you in the victim role. Instead, reframe your thinking in a more positive and empowering way: "I choose not to eat that cake because I don't want to."

So how do you get out of this victim mindset?

Remind yourself every day that you hold the power to make decisions that will either move you toward your goals or move you away from them. Whether you stick to your fasting goals or eat processed foods is up to you and nobody else.

You also have to learn to set boundaries both for yourself and for other people. It's OK to say no to food even when other people are eating and when they don't agree with you and what you're doing.

Stop People-Pleasing and Do Instead of Try

I used to be a huge people pleaser, and to an extent, maybe I still am. Change is an ongoing process. But finally losing weight and getting to my goal weight *required* me to come to terms with this part of myself. When you put other people's needs, wants, and opinions above your own, you're shooting yourself in the foot. Trying to make *everyone* happy won't make *anyone* happy—least of all you. You need to start focusing on *you*, and sometimes that involves upsetting a few people along the way.

Finally, stop telling yourself that you'll try: "I'll try to make it to a twenty-four-hour fast" or "I'll try to stay keto at the restaurant." Do or don't on this journey; there is no try. Make a decision that you're ready for and lock it in. When you allow yourself to "try," you leave the door open for negotiation and failure. In effect, you're telling yourself that you don't believe in your ability to make it to your goal. Changing how you talk to yourself is crucial for your success—so change your *I'll try* to *I will*.

Sit with It

When you're fasting, you'll sometimes have uncomfortable feelings and thoughts—hunger pangs, cravings, nausea, weakness, or thoughts of giving in and eating a bunch of high-sugar, high-carb foods. It's OK to have uncomfortable thoughts and feelings. The key is to be mindful of how you *respond* to those thoughts and feelings. Thoughts can't hurt you unless you decide to act on them in a negative way. It's fine to feel scared, anxious, or like you want to give up, but just because you're feeling or thinking something doesn't mean that you have to impulsively act on it.

Sometimes, uncomfortable feelings can make you want to run away from them or numb them, and a lot of the time, you might want to turn to food. But it's important not to use food as a coping or numbing mechanism for uncomfortable feelings.

The next time you have an uncomfortable feeling, try just sitting with it. Observe the feelings and let them be there with you. Allow yourself to fully feel them and experience them. But make sure you don't white-knuckle your way through the thoughts. Relax and try to let them go. Once you have acknowledged them and breathed through them, chances are that they'll pass on their own.

If they don't pass, reflect on why you're feeling the way you are or having those thoughts. Do you have any underlying stressors in your life? Are you feeling anxious about something? If those things are happening, you can take actions to deal with the underlying causes.

And if you aren't anxious or stressed about other things but your uncomfortable feelings and thoughts aren't going away, that's OK too. You can allow them to be there with you without doing anything about them. Just like a lot of other things in life that exist and are unpleasant but don't have a solution (like taxes or unpicked-up dog poop), you have to accept your feelings' existence and then move on with your life.

Separate the craving from the *action*. Allowing yourself to sit with the discomfort helps you train yourself because these feelings won't last forever, even though it might seem like it right now. Every time you get a craving, consider it an opportunity to get stronger. The more you resist giving in to your cravings or uncomfortable feelings in these times, the easier it will become to resist them in the future.

It's OK to be uncomfortable. It's OK to have hard feelings. It's OK to have cravings or to think that fasting is really difficult. That doesn't mean you have to give up.

You have to get comfortable with being uncomfortable because real growth happens outside of your comfort zone. I'm not suggesting you have to accept living a hard life, but instead of viewing every challenge as a negative, view it as a chance to improve yourself.

The life you want is on the other side of your comfort zone, so you have to push yourself to get there. Staying within your comfort zone is what got you to where you are now: uncomfortable, overweight, and full of inflammation. You have the power to change that, but you have to take the leap. Feeling uncomfortable is a sign that you're making progress; you're growing and pushing past all the things that you thought you couldn't handle. Your dream life lies on the other side of that discomfort, so if you're feeling uncomfortable, you know you're on the right track.

Love Yourself Through It

You need to stop criticizing yourself and thinking that being "perfect" is all that matters. Instead, you need to have a huge amount of love and compassion for yourself. As I've said before, you can't hate yourself into becoming a version of yourself that you love. You also can't hate yourself into achieving your goal weight.

Hating yourself never works because as soon as you hit a roadblock, and there will be several, hate won't be able to get you through it. When you're struggling, hate only causes you to have more negative thoughts, which push you further into your unhealthy habits and further away from achieving your goals. When you come across challenges or struggle to stay on track or stay motivated, make sure that you show yourself so much love that you have no other choice but to carry on.

When you have a slip, the first step is to forgive yourself. There will be times when you don't stay on plan or when you make decisions that don't align with your ultimate goal. These moments are not failures; they're part of being human. Beating yourself up only leads to a cycle of negativity that will stop your progress. So forgive yourself for the mistake and release yourself from any shame, guilt, or negativity that's tied to it. The sooner you can unshackle yourself from the negative action, the sooner you can move on. If you don't cut that tie, you're going to stay attached to your mistake, and it's going to end up dragging you under. You don't want that. Acknowledge the slip, forgive yourself, learn from it, and get back on track.

No matter what mistake you've made, there's always an opportunity for you to learn something from it. I recommend that my clients use a mistake as a journaling topic. Write about what happened and why it happened, and then think about ways you can prevent it from happening in the future.

Loving yourself also involves celebrating yourself when you complete your everyday tasks and habits. You might not notice huge changes or be crossing huge milestones all the time, but no matter how little progress you're making, you're still moving forward, and that deserves to be celebrated.

Did you make it through a fasting period without giving in to your cravings? That's a win. Did you manage to choose keto foods over high-carb, highly processed snacks last night? Another win. Did you lose one ounce on the scale this morning? That's another win! All these things are milestones. No matter how small and insignificant they may seem, they're all achievements that lead you closer to your goal weight. So whether a small win is a weight-loss victory or a nonscale victory, make sure you give yourself love for it. Major progress is made up of hundreds of tiny steps along the way, so it's important not to ignore them.

If you have a hard time loving yourself, I want you to pick one thing—just one thing—that you love about yourself right now. Actually, I'll up the stakes. Pick one thing you love about yourself and one thing you love about your *body*. The thing you love about yourself can be how caring you are to your friends and family, or it can be the fact that you showed up for yourself today even if you didn't want to. Even if you don't like where your body is right now, there must still be something you like about it. It can be your wrists or your eyelashes, for all I care—but pick something and love yourself for it. Do this every day, and you'll start to build a loving and positive view of yourself, which will help you achieve so much more success on this journey.

Handle the Scale

The scale can be your friend, but it can also be your worst enemy. If you know how to use it correctly, it can be a powerful tool in helping you get to your goals.

The scale objectively tells you whether you're making progress, but when you're going up and down in weight and you don't know why, it can drive you nuts. Because the scale can be unpredictable, it's very easy to get hooked on it and let it mess with your mood and self-image. So you need to use the scale as a tool to help you without letting it hurt you along the way.

KEEP YOUR FEELINGS OUT OF IT

Don't get too emotionally attached to the number on the scale or attach your happiness or self-worth to it. I know that this is easier said than done, but step one in this game, as you know, is mindset. Instead of filling yourself with dread over stepping on the scale and letting it control how you feel, try to reframe your thinking. See the scale as a simple tool for data collection. With each weigh-in, you collect a new data point on a very long graph. Think of it in terms of scientific research. Each data point is not very helpful on its own, but once you collect enough data points, you'll be able to see patterns that will help you determine whether you're moving in the right direction.

WEIGH ONCE A DAY

I usually suggest weighing every day. The purpose is not to nitpick on yourself but to gather information. Weighing every day enables you to track changes over time and gives you a clearer overview of your body's fluctuations.

It's totally normal for your weight to fluctuate slightly day to day, especially for women. Hormones and cycles can affect how much water women carry on their bodies, which shows up on the scale.

Weighing yourself often allows you to track these weight fluctuations over time and understand what's causing them. Weekly weigh-ins can give you an inaccurate picture of your progress. Let's say Monday morning is your weekly weigh-in day, and your weight is 200 pounds. During the week, your weight goes down to 198 on Tuesday, 196 on Thursday, 197 on Sunday, and on Monday you're up to 200 pounds again because you're carrying a little bit of extra water weight due to your cycle. If you weigh only once a week (on Monday), all you're seeing is that you lost no weight at all that week, despite all your hard work. You can become disheartened and feel like what you're doing isn't working. But in actual fact, you lost 4 pounds that week, and the scale will likely reflect that in another couple of days.

When you weigh in every day, you can keep track of the downward trend, despite the daily fluctuations. And when you understand that weight fluctuations are all part of the process, and even expected, you're less likely to let a temporary increase on the scale weigh you down. Pardon the pun!

LEARN FROM THE DATA

Once you have used the scale for a while, you'll be able to track how your weight has changed over time and see how your body responds to different foods, activities, and your cycle. For example, you may find that you're sensitive to a specific food that stalls your weight loss or notice that your weight follows a pattern throughout the month. You can choose not to have that specific food anymore or relax in the knowledge that your weight is up because of where you are in the monthly pattern.

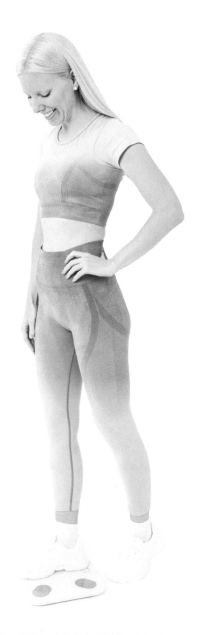

The scale is a tool—no more, no less. The data from the scale can help you make decisions that lead to weight loss but only when you use it wisely. When you view weighing as data collection but don't use it to judge yourself, you can keep a healthy and balanced relationship with the scale. (Another scale pun—I'm on a roll!)

CHAPTER 11
BREAKING BAD (HABITS)

You probably don't realize that the way you're living your life is causing a bunch of inflammation in your body. Chronic inflammation can be the cause of many problems, such as weight gain, tiredness, and even severe conditions like heart disease, diabetes, and autoimmune diseases. In this chapter, I explain how your current bad habits promote inflammation and ways you can break those habits.

UNDERSTANDING the CONNECTION BETWEEN INFLAMMATION and EATING and LIFESTYLE HABITS

To be able to break the bad habits that cause inflammation, you need to know the specific things you're doing that contribute to the problem. In this section, I cover many of the common causes of inflammation.

Eating Processed Foods

One of the biggest contributors to inflammation is eating highly processed, high-carb foods. These foods are staples of the standard Western diet and are loaded with sugars, refined grains, and processed fats that can trigger inflammatory responses in your body. Unlike whole foods, which are rich in nutrients that are beneficial for your health, processed foods are often completely lacking in them. To lower your inflammation, you should stick to a diet low in carbs and stay away from processed foods and seed oils. Adding fiber and apple cider vinegar to your diet can also help reduce inflammation.

Constantly Eating

Our bodies are built to cycle between feasting and fasting, but modern habits have completely disrupted this system because we are constantly snacking and eating throughout the day. We hardly give our bodies a break. Eating frequently, especially when what we eat is a diet high in heavily processed foods, can lead to high blood sugar and insulin resistance, which are both linked with increased inflammation. Also, eating in this way can disrupt the balance of hunger hormones, causing more inflammation and weight gain.

Living a Highly Stressed Life

Stress can come from a variety of places, such as your work, your personal life, or even exercise, and these heightened stress levels increase inflammation. The chronic stress caused by modern-day living keeps your body in a constant state of alert, which leads to constant release of stress hormones, such as cortisol. Cortisol in itself is not a harmful hormone, and it's useful in acutely stressful situations, but too much cortisol can harm your immune system and promote inflammation.[1]

Working out too intensely can also cause an increased stress response, something a lot of people are surprised to hear. I've stopped doing high-intensity interval training (HIIT) and other high-intensity workouts at the gym because I felt that it was stressing me out and causing anxiety, so now I stick to low-intensity exercise, like walking and anything that I can do while still remaining calm.

Drinking Sweet and Low-Calorie Drinks

Drinks with sugar or artificial sweeteners can be a hidden source of inflammation in the body. Drinking sugary drinks, and even diet drinks, will lead to spikes in insulin levels and contribute to an inflammatory environment in your body.[2] Although diet drinks don't have any calories, the artificial sweetener in these drinks can disrupt your gut microbiome, which has been identified as a key cause in developing chronic inflammation.[3]

Not Getting Enough Sleep

Sleep is crucially important for your health, but it's easy to forget about sleep when you're leading a busy life. Not sleeping enough can have major impacts on your body, making inflammation worse. When you're sleeping, your body goes through a variety of repair processes, including regulating and controlling inflammation in your body. Not having enough sleep disrupts these processes and causes inflammation, which increases your risk of developing a variety of inflammatory-related diseases.[4]

BREAKING the BINGE CYCLE

A lot of people struggle with binge eating. You might be one of those people. If you eat loads of food quickly and end up feeling out of control or that you're completely controlled by your cravings, you might have a binge-eating problem. Binge eating completely derails your journey when you're trying to lose weight and get healthy.

Also, bingeing often leads to a binge-and-restrict cycle, which is when you've binged and then you try to overcompensate by severely restricting your calories, overexercising, or fasting. But this cycle of bingeing and restricting is not just incredibly harmful to your physical health but also to your mental well-being. Understanding what causes bingeing and repairing your mindset around food are crucial steps toward breaking this cycle and achieving a healthier relationship with food.

What Causes Binge Eating?

Overeating or bingeing is not only about physical hunger; it's a psychological compulsion. You feel an overwhelming urge to eat, often as a response to emotional triggers rather than actual hunger. A lot of things can trigger binge eating, including emotional stress, restrictive dieting, negative body issues, hormonal issues, and excessive food obsession. Emotional triggers can make you turn to food for comfort. Eating is a coping mechanism to deal with negative feelings in the same way using alcohol or drugs is a coping mechanism for an alcoholic or a drug addict.

Because the causes of binge eating are emotional rather than physical, indulging in binge-eating behavior usually leads to feelings of guilt and shame, which can trigger a compulsion to restrict food intake to make up for the binge. But this behavior only keeps the binge-restrict cycle going, so it's important for you to break free from this way of thinking.

Hormonal imbalances, and especially those that affect hunger and fullness cues, can also cause binge-eating behaviors. Understanding the underlying causes of binge eating is the first step to beating it.

Overcoming Emotional Eating and Food Cravings

To stop binge eating, you need to change how you think and move away from a mindset of restriction and guilt to a mindset of mindfulness and self-compassion. Here are some ways you can do so:

- **Identify your triggers and emotional eating patterns:** The most important thing you can do is identify what emotional or environmental triggers lead you to binge-eat. Keep a food and mood journal to help you pinpoint patterns in your behavior and emotions so that you can see which feelings and situations trigger binge episodes.

- **Practice mindfulness and mindful eating:** Eating mindfully helps prevent bingeing. Focus on the taste, texture, and pleasure of food without any distractions. Eating mindfully helps you to listen to your true hunger and fullness cues, which reduces the likelihood of overeating.

- **Stop restrictive dieting:** Restrictive dieting, such as calorie counting or following an exact meal plan, can give you a lot of stress and anxiety related to food. Try to adopt a more flexible approach to your eating, making sure that you eat a wide variety of low-carb and nutrient-dense foods, such as meat, fish, green vegetables, and loads of healthy fats.

- **Create coping strategies:** Because binge eating is often caused by emotionally triggering situations, you need to find healthy coping mechanisms to handle your stress. Exercising, journaling, meditating, or talking with a friend can help keep you distracted and offer some emotional support without the need to turn to food.

- **Self-compassion:** Always be kind to yourself and remind yourself that struggles are a normal part of weight loss. Instead of punishing yourself after a binge, try to understand why it happened and what you can learn from the experience so you can avoid putting yourself in that situation in the future.

- **Know when to get expert help:** Sometimes, the cycle of binge eating and restricting can be too tough to handle by yourself. If that's the case, going to see a therapist or somebody who specializes in managing eating issues can help provide you with specific methods to help you overcome binge-eating behaviors.

CUTTING OUT ALCOHOL

Drinking alcohol is something a lot of people enjoy, but it can really affect both your health and your weight-loss efforts in a negative way. I've almost completely cut alcohol out of my life, and I feel so much better for it. To be successful on your weight-loss journey, you need to understand how alcohol can lead to inflammation, water retention, and weight-loss stalls.

Alcohol and Inflammation

When you have an injury or infection, your body reacts by creating inflammation as part of the healing process. But as I mentioned in other chapters, chronic inflammation can lead to health issues such as heart disease, diabetes, and obesity, so you want to avoid doing things that worsen the inflammation. Drinking alcohol is one of those things.

Why does alcohol consumption trigger an inflammation response in your body? Because alcohol is broken down into a substance called acetaldehyde, which is a toxic chemical that can damage the tissues in the body.[5] When acetaldehyde is present in your body, it tells your immune system to respond with inflammation. If you drink on a regular basis, it can lead to chronic inflammation, which can make existing health issues worse and keep your body from working at its best.

Alcohol and Water Retention

Water retention, or carrying excess water weight, is another side effect of drinking alcohol that can impact your weight and health. Alcohol can cause dehydration, which makes your body hold on to water to maintain fluid balance. The result is a bloated feeling and puffiness, especially in your hands, feet, and face. And, of course, carrying excess water weight also shows up on the scale.

On top of this, drinking alcohol can throw off your electrolytes, which can make water retention and bloating even worse and slow your weight-loss progress.

Alcohol and Weight Loss

Alcohol affects weight loss in several ways. Alcoholic drinks are often high in calories and low in nutrients, which means that drinking alcohol can increase your calorie intake without giving you any essential vitamins and minerals. When you drink alcohol, you're more likely to make bad food choices and eat too much. This is because drinking alcohol can mess with your judgment and increases your hunger. Just think of the number of times you've gone to a fast-food joint after a night out and eaten way more unhealthily than you should have.

Another crucial point is that alcohol slows down your body's ability to burn fat because your body prioritizes breaking down alcohol before it breaks down anything else. As a result, your body won't be able to break down body fat until it's broken down and burned off all the alcohol first, so drinking alcohol severely slows down your weight-loss efforts.

Finally, alcohol can negatively affect your sleep. Not having enough sleep makes you feel more tired the next day, meaning you're less likely to make good food choices. Sleep deprivation has also been shown to cause you to eat more calories than you do after you've had a good night's sleep.[6]

Drinking alcohol is harmful to your body and should be something that you try to cut down, if not eliminate completely. If possible during your weight-loss journey, I recommend that you cut out alcohol completely to see the biggest benefits.

If you're unable or unwilling to cut out alcohol, there are certain things to think about if you want to stay on track with your weight-loss goals. The first is to cut out all sugary alcoholic drinks and cocktails. Stick to dry wines and hard liquors, such as vodka, tequila, and whiskey. One of my favorite go-to cocktails back when I was drinking on a keto lifestyle was vodka soda with a slice of lime. The second thing is to limit your alcohol intake as much as you can.

Bad habits like eating processed foods, binge eating, and consuming alcohol can wreak havoc on your body, so it's important to swap them for better habits that support a healthier and happier life going forward. In the next chapter, I discuss how to properly refeed after fasting to prevent regaining weight and ensure that you keep reaping the benefits of fasting and weight loss for the rest of your life.

CHAPTER 12

BREAKING YOUR FAST CORRECTLY: THE CRUCIAL FACTOR IN WEIGHT LOSS

It's important that you break your fast properly to give your body a chance to recover from the fast. It's also important to always have some foods ready in case you need to break your fast unexpectedly. Being prepared with the right types of food prevents you from breaking your fast with food that can potentially undo your progress or, worse, harm your health. So make sure you refeed slowly with soft and nutrient-dense foods to keep you safe and healthy.

In this chapter, I go over some general guidelines for how to refeed safely after a fast, how to deal with breaking a fast sooner than expected, why you should avoid sweeteners, and how simple diet hacks can increase your fat-burning.

GENERAL REFEEDING GUIDELINES

How you break a fast is sometimes even more important to the success of the fast than the fast itself. The way you break your fast is ultimately up to you, but breaking safely prevents you from completely undoing all the progress you have made on your fast.

Also, refeeding safely and carefully prevents you from developing potentially dangerous side effects such as refeeding syndrome and edema, both of which are caused by breaking a fast with foods that are high in carbohydrates or eating proteins too soon after a long fast. You have already done many great things for your body by completing a fast, so make sure you keep it up by refeeding safely.

WHAT IS REFEEDING SYNDROME?

Refeeding syndrome can occur when there's a sudden shift in electrolytes that help your body process food, and this can happen after long periods without food.[1] When you're fasting, your insulin levels stay extremely low. When you reintroduce food after a long time of fasting, your body has to quickly shift from burning your body fat for fuel to burning glucose for fuel, and insulin levels increase. If insulin levels are increased too high or too quickly, it can be a shock to the system.

There are many symptoms of refeeding syndrome, including weakness, dizziness, breathing difficulties, high blood pressure, seizures, coma, and death. The symptoms of refeeding syndrome typically occur within the first couple of days of refeeding. To prevent refeeding syndrome, it's important to keep insulin levels as low as possible in your refeed to slowly reintroduce your body to metabolizing food. Never consume high-carb or high-sugar foods after a long fast. Keto foods have very little effect on your insulin, which is why your refeed should always be strict keto. If you are experiencing any of the listed symptoms or are at all worried that you might be experiencing refeeding syndrome, seek immediate medical attention.

During your refeed, stay away from high-carb and processed foods. If you've done a long extended fast (for example, a week or longer), also make sure you stay away from anything crunchy or hard, which can hurt or scratch your intestines. You want to be as kind as possible to your digestive system. If you're coming off a shorter fast, you can be a lot more lenient with the types of foods and textures you eat as long as you follow the general guidelines of eating slowly and sticking to a low-carb diet. With a longer fast, you should stick to soft green vegetables like salads or broccoli in the first few days of refeeding.

Breaking a Short Fast

In this section, I explain the general guidelines for breaking fasts of one to three days.

FASTS OF TWENTY-FOUR HOURS OR LESS

Fasts that are twenty-four hours or shorter don't usually require any specific refeeding guidelines or procedures for breaking your fast, but you should still take care to gently break your fast. When you break your fast, you may be tempted to eat a lot of food, but it's important that you try to avoid this urge.

Most people experience psychological hunger rather than physical hunger as the time to break a fast approaches, so make sure you're being careful and taking steps to avoid overeating. Even when breaking a short fast, eating too much can cause stomach pain, which isn't usually dangerous, but it can be very uncomfortable. It's important to focus on eating only until you're satisfied rather than stuffed or overly full. Make sure that you drink plenty of water and stick to keto foods such as eggs; fatty cuts of meats such as beef, chicken, or fish; and green above-ground vegetables such as broccoli, cauliflower, lettuce, and avocado.

TWO- OR THREE-DAY FASTS

Breaking a fast that's lasted two or three days requires you to be a little bit more careful. Always wait until you're truly hungry before breaking your fast. When you decide to have something, I recommend starting with a small amount of bone broth or a clear soup. Feel free to enhance it with butter, cream, or oil. You can also add heavy cream to your coffee or tea. After that, you can have a small to medium-sized meal such as some soft-boiled eggs, avocado, steamed cauliflower or broccoli, and a soft protein like chicken or fish.

Always take care to eat slowly, and never eat until the point where you're feeling stuffed. Stop at the point where you're just satisfied. As long as everything has gone smoothly after you eat your first meal, you can proceed with regular keto meals, being mindful not to overeat.

Breaking an Extended Fast

When breaking an extended fast of more than three days, it's important to make sure you're doing so safely. Breaking a long fast improperly can result in not only uncomfortable side effects such as diarrhea, nausea, and stomachaches but also serious health complications, including refeeding syndrome, which is a dangerous and potentially fatal condition that can occur if food is introduced too quickly or improperly after a long period without food.

As long as you follow the refeeding guidelines, you'll keep yourself safe and won't have to worry about any dangerous side effects. If you've been fasting for several days or longer, it's important to keep taking your electrolytes during your refeed to ensure your mineral levels stay balanced. The electrolytes will help you avoid uncomfortable side effects such as headaches and dehydration. It is also advised that you take a vitamin B supplement and a phosphorus supplement around thirty minutes before breaking your fast. Do this before each meal during the complete length of your refeed, which should be around half of the length of your fast. For example, if you fast for seven days, your refeed should be around three days; if you fasted for ten days, your refeed should be around five days.

SEVEN- TO TEN-DAY FASTS

After a seven- to ten-day fast, you should plan to refeed for four to five days while continuing to take your electrolytes. Here's a general outline of how to handle your refeed:

DAY 1

After any length of fast, make sure you start your day with plenty of water to help your digestive system. Use this day to get used to eating again and limit overeating. You can add butter or heavy cream to your coffee or tea. On the first day, I recommend eating pureed soups, such as broccoli or cauliflower, and mashed avocado with sea salt and lemon.

DAY 2

On the second day after breaking your fast, you can start to introduce soft steamed keto vegetables, salads, soft-boiled eggs, and small amounts of cheese. Make sure you eat foods with a high fat content, and always stick to strict keto foods.

DAY 3

Keep following the feeding instructions from Day 2, but you can start to slowly increase the quantity of food. Still always make sure you eat only until you're satisfied, not stuffed. You can also start to introduce some soft proteins, such as fish or chicken. Low-carb fish or chicken soup is great for Day 3.

DAY 4

On this day, you can eat regular serving sizes of anything I mentioned for Days 1 through 3, and you can also start to introduce any additional keto foods of your choice.

FOURTEEN-DAY FASTS

For a fourteen-day fast, plan to refeed for a full seven days and keep taking your electrolytes. Here's my suggested refeeding schedule:

DAY 1

Avocado, bone broth, bulletproof coffee (coffee mixed with butter), and coffee with heavy cream are great ways to start breaking your fourteen-day fast. After that, make sure you wait at least an hour or until you're truly hungry; then you can choose a small serving of keto vegetables, such as pureed cauliflower or broccoli. Add salt and butter to make sure you're keeping both your electrolyte and fat intake levels high.

DAY 2

Continue to eat any of the items from Day 1, and you can also start to add soft-boiled eggs at the end of Day 2 as long as you're feeling good and haven't experienced any digestive issues from anything you've already eaten.

DAY 3

Continue eating as you have on Days 1 and 2, but you can also add cheese and more fresh leafy greens.

DAYS 4 TO 6

For the next three days, you can eat everything previously mentioned, but you can have larger amounts as long as you're not overeating. Always make sure that you keep your carbohydrate intake low (less than 20 grams). What carbs you do eat should come from green vegetables. Eating too many carbs at this point can make you feel unwell or cause you to struggle with thoughts of overeating. At this point, you can also start to introduce soft animal proteins, such as fish and chicken, but always make sure that you're keeping your portion sizes small because your stomach won't be used to full servings.

DAY 7

On the last day of your refeed, you should start to make the switch to a regular keto diet. You should be back to eating full-sized meals while making sure that you eat only until you're satisfied rather than stuffed. Keep the fat content high and the carb content low to manage your appetite.

Although seven days might seem like a long time to refeed after a fourteen-day fast, refeeding gradually and gently has many benefits. You're less likely to overeat, and you're also less likely to have serious digestive issues. Refeeding slowly and gently also helps you tune in to your body's true hunger and fullness cues, so you can keep track of how your body reacts to different types of foods.

TWENTY-ONE-DAY FASTS

After a twenty-one-day fast, plan to refeed for a full ten days and continue to take your electrolytes.

DAY 1

Bone broth, avocado, bulletproof coffee, and coffee with heavy cream are all excellent ways to start breaking your fast. You can also prepare low-carb vegetable juice made from keto vegetables and diluted with water. Wait at least an hour before eating anything solid. When you do introduce solids, have pureed low-carb vegetables such as broccoli or cauliflower.

DAY 2

This day repeats Day 1, but you can start including soft-boiled eggs and a slightly thicker soup made from low-carb vegetables. Make sure you eat slowly, and only introduce eggs if you haven't had any digestive issues up until this point. If you have experienced issues with digestion, such as stomach pain, bloating, or diarrhea, it's best to hold off on eggs until Day 3.

DAYS 3 TO 4

On these two days, continue as you have been, but include eggs and cheese. You can also start to introduce more green watery vegetables, such as cucumbers and soft leafy salads.

DAYS 5 TO 7

You can eat larger amounts of the foods mentioned in Days 1 through 4. Make sure you keep your carbohydrate levels, which should come only from keto vegetable sources, below 20 grams per day. Too many carbs at this point can put you at risk for trigger overeating. You can have soft and easily digestible proteins, such as fish or chicken, but make sure you start with only small amounts to check how well you tolerate them before you continue with higher amounts.

DAYS 8 TO 10

Full-fat dairy is on the table in addition to any of the foods previously mentioned. Use these days to slowly increase your portion sizes if you need to, but remember to eat only until satisfied—never stuffed. Don't force yourself to eat if you're not hungry, and never force yourself to finish a meal if you feel satisfied before you've eaten all of it.

Refeeding for ten days may seem like a long time to end a three-week fast, but a slow refeed ensures that you keep reaping the benefits of your fast. Taking things slowly means you're less likely to undo all the progress you've made through your fast. You're also less likely to have digestive issues, and refeeding slowly can help you become more aware of your body's hunger and fullness cues. Think of the refeed as a tool to change your relationship to food going forward.

FASTS OF THIRTY DAYS OR MORE

If you've been fasting for thirty days or more, a slow refeed is crucial. Slowly refeeding after such a long fast ensures that you keep yourself safe and protect yourself from developing refeeding syndrome or other serious health complications. Always approach a long fast like this with caution.

DAY 1

You can start to break your fast with bone broth, bulletproof coffee, or coffee with cream. You can add butter, cream, or oil to your bone broth. You can make a vegetable juice of up to 50 percent keto vegetables and at least 50 percent water. Keep drinking these liquids every few hours throughout the first day. Do not introduce solids on Day 1 because they can lead to digestive issues.

DAY 2

Repeat the protocol from Day 1 for the first half of the day. If things have been going well, you haven't experienced any digestive issues, and you feel ready to eat solid food, you can try having some avocado or pureed keto vegetables, such as broccoli or cauliflower. Make sure you add butter and salt for flavor, electrolytes, and fat. The solid foods you eat should be soft and easy to digest because having hard or crunchy foods prematurely might scratch or damage your intestines.

DAYS 3 TO 4

At this point, you can introduce slightly heavier and thicker soups, and you can keep having servings of pureed broccoli or cauliflower and mashed avocado with sea salt and lemon. During this time, you can also start to add soft-boiled eggs if you've been handling the other foods well without experiencing any problems with digestion.

DAYS 5 TO 6

Keep eating the previously mentioned foods, including eggs, and start to add leafy vegetables and cucumbers. You can also eat some cheese. Only eat until you're satisfied but not stuffed. It's important to use this time to refeed slowly and prevent overeating.

DAYS 7 TO 8

After a week of refeeding, you can slowly increase the portion sizes of the foods you've been eating. You can also start introducing soft and easily digested proteins such as chicken or fish. Make sure that you keep your daily carbohydrate intake below 20 grams per day, with all of your carbs coming from green above-ground vegetables. Consuming too many carbs can trigger overeating, so it's important that you're careful about this.

DAYS 9 TO 15

For the last several days of your refeed, you can introduce full-fat dairy and more types of keto vegetables. Use these days to transition into your regular keto diet. By Day 15, you should be back to eating regular-sized meals, although you should still eat only until you're satisfied. As I mentioned earlier, the fast should be a way to change your relationship with food, which includes changing your portion sizes. Most people gain weight because they have an unhealthy relationship to food, including the amount of food they eat. Eating less, as long as you feel satisfied, is totally fine and will help you maintain the benefits of your fast.

Although 15 days might seem like a long time to break a fast, breaking slowly makes you less likely to be triggered to overeat. You're also less likely to have digestive issues. Refeeding slowly helps you tune in to your hunger and fullness cues and reduces the risk that you'll develop serious health complications.

You can use the general guidelines I've offered for refeeding, but always listen to your body. If anything feels wrong or if you're not tolerating certain foods, go slower. If you're ever worried about your health or well-being, always consult a medical professional.

WHAT to DO if YOU BREAK YOUR FAST EARLY

If you end up breaking your fast earlier than you planned, you can easily start down a negative spiral and feel like you've had a huge setback on your fasting journey. Remember, though, achieving your goals isn't a straight line, and there will inevitably be ups and downs. How you handle these ups and downs determines how successful you are in the long term.

Unguilt Yourself

When you end up breaking a fast earlier than planned—whether it's because of unforeseen circumstances or giving in to excuses—it's important not to guilt yourself too much for it. Everybody struggles sometimes, and it's common not to be successful right away. The goal is not to be perfect but to make progress. So if you break your fast too early, acknowledge that you broke it and think about why you did, but try not to judge yourself too harshly for it.

How you respond to breaking your fast early is the most important factor. Get out of the perfection mindset where you tell yourself that you're either doing perfectly or you're going to throw it all out the window. This all-or-nothing way of thinking only makes you feel guilty, and it's not serving you. Try to let go of that mindset and realize that one slip neither defines you nor undoes all the progress you've made. The sooner you can get out of that mindset, the sooner you can get back on track and feel good again.

Don't Overcompensate if You Overeat or Fall Off Track

When you've broken your fast too early—especially if you broke it with something less than ideal, like chocolate cake or a full-on food binge—you can easily slide into a mindset where you try to overcompensate for the slip by committing to an even lengthier fast or overexercising. But this way of thinking is harmful and can put you at risk for a really unhealthy binge-and-restrict cycle that can be very difficult to break free of. So instead of overcompensating, try to move on and get back to your regular fasting schedule as quickly as you can. Trust the process: One day or one slip will not ruin your whole journey. The most important thing is that you build consistency over time without using extreme measures to deal with what is actually a minor setback in the big picture of your journey.

Reset After a Binge

Breaking your fast too early can sometimes lead to a binge, where you eat large amounts of food out of guilt or compensation for other negative feelings. If you find yourself in a binge after breaking your fast too early, it's really important to approach the situation with a calm mindset, where you focus on learning and understanding rather than punishing yourself.

First off, think about why you binged and write the reason down on paper. Check in with yourself: Were you extra stressed for some reason? Did you have any triggering foods around you? Were you part of triggering events or around triggering people? What were the exact excuses you told yourself to convince yourself that it was OK to go off plan?

Be completely honest with yourself. Take some time to journal about it because doing so helps you identify and understand your individual triggers, which will help you avoid putting yourself in those situations in the future or, at the very least, help you develop healthier coping mechanisms for yourself in those situations.

Right after a binge, it's also important to focus on hydrating properly and nourishing your body with balanced and healthy foods. Make sure you drink a large glass of water to signal the end of the binge. For your next meal, make sure you have healthy, nutritious, low-carb food to stabilize your blood sugar levels and nourish your body properly.

Resetting after a binge should never be about restricting but about caring for yourself properly, both mentally and physically.

Return to your regular planned fasting schedule—whether that's an extended fast or an intermittent fast—as quickly as you can. Make sure you pick up where you left off. Resisting the urge to "make up" for the binge by fasting longer helps you break the binge-and-restrict cycle and helps you develop a healthier relationship to food and your fasting routine.

It's also important to forgive yourself. Neither fasting nor working to lose weight is easy. On this fasting-for-weight-loss journey, you're not just going through a physical transformation but also a mental transformation, and that can be really tough sometimes. So it's important that you recognize how hard you're working and not let one small setback derail your whole journey.

Use the Experience as a Learning Opportunity

Breaking a fast early is a learning opportunity. It doesn't automatically mean you've failed. When you break your fast earlier than intended, it's a great opportunity to learn about yourself and grow on your fasting journey. Every step of the way, you're building your muscle and moving the needle, even if you don't always feel like it. The more you learn and the more you grow, the easier this journey will become for you.

CLIENT SPOTLIGHT: ERIN

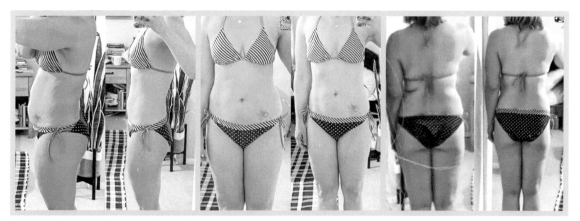

STARTING WEIGHT	149.4 lbs
CURRENT WEIGHT	124.8 lbs
TOTAL WEIGHT LOST	24.6 lbs

I've been on a weight-loss journey for twelve years, and I've tried several different ways to lose weight. Anytime I would try a new diet, I would feel almost excited at first. I would do a lot of planning and meal prepping, but eventually it would become a drag and unsustainable because of all the rules and the work involved, not to mention the extra time and money.

What I like about fasting is that it's simple. Unlike other diets, where rules seemed to govern every meal, fasting boiled down to a binary choice: Eat or don't eat. And even though I might not be eating right now, I know that it's only temporary, and I can have tacos later. So that knowledge provides a level of sanity and peace of mind.

Eventually, I got into a pretty good rhythm with fasting, but it was definitely a journey to get there. At first, I struggled to prioritize long-term goals over momentary cravings, but I realized that any feelings of hunger or cravings only lasted ten minutes. Instead of my hunger getting worse and worse, like I thought it would, it would literally just go away. All I had to do was distract myself with a quick activity—something like a brief walk.

Another thing I struggled with was fasting during a social event, but once I realized the extent to which humans eat on autopilot (we eat because it's 7:00 p.m., we eat because something awesome happened, we eat because something bad happened, and so on), I realized how much emotion and mindlessness is tied to eating, and it made me want to be above it.

Fortunately, fasting is super flexible. I utilized the different options of daily intermittent fasting, alternate-day fasting, and longer extended fasts. This allowed fasting to fit into my life in a way that accommodated not only my goals, but anything else I had going on, like a vacation, a wedding, or a concert. By flexing my "mental toughness" muscle (and feeling pretty smug while doing it), I even fasted through social events. But I've also planned ahead and stacked the front of my week with longer fasts so that I could take a day off at the end of the week. I realized I was in the driver's seat, so I took charge and made fasting work for me.

There were little issues along the way, like the first time I did an extended fast. I encountered mild restless leg symptoms in the evenings. A simple internet search cleared up the source of the issue, and I started making sure I was taking in more electrolytes. Situations like this make me think of the phrase, "Either way is hard. Pick your hard." So yes, fasting was hard at first, but I realized that the struggles that came with fasting were only momentary, and they fortunately came with quick solutions like increasing electrolytes to eliminate restless legs. But the other "hard"—for example, the "hard" that came with squeezing into a shirt that was too tight and walking around all day feeling uncomfortable—that "hard" didn't come with a quick fix. Sure, I could buy a bigger shirt, but being of short stature, bigger clothes swallow me up. And what if it's hot, and I want to wear a tank top without my chubby arms flapping around? It became so clear to me that fasting was the easier "hard" option!

Finding fasting not only meant I was losing weight, but I began to generalize the mindset of mental toughness and delayed gratification to other areas of life, which I loved doing! I continued to embrace fasting and evolve my view of it. I began to see fasting not as a lack of something or avoidance of something but rather as an embracing of something, specifically my goals in life. For me, fasting was the result of reprioritizing the things I truly wanted in the long run. And what I want in the long run was not a quick bite to eat that I wouldn't even think about again ten minutes after I finish it. I also began to love how fasting gave me back time and money, once again showing me that fasting isn't a lack of something. It's abundance!

At this point, fasting has been a part of my life for more than a year. Not only has fasting helped me to lose weight and maintain the weight loss, but it's helped me to become more picky with what I put in my body. If I'm only eating one meal on a particular day, for example, I'm going to make sure it's a meal that is worthy and will nourish my body. I think my favorite thing since beginning fasting is that it has snapped me out of the societal norms of eating. My eating isn't on autopilot. For example, my husband and I don't automatically prepare and eat dinner every night. We check in with each other. Maybe one of us had a late lunch and isn't hungry. Maybe we only feel like something light. So fasting has brought about a greater level of intentionality to my eating.

Looking back now, I can see that fasting was a journey of self-discovery and empowerment for me. Through its simplicity, adaptability, and transformative potential, fasting has not only reshaped my body but also changed my perspective on day-to-day life.

DON'T EAT CARBS on their OWN

I am under no illusion that your weight-loss journey will have its ups and downs, and it's unrealistic to think that you're always going to be perfect when it comes to food choices.

When you find yourself in a situation where you eat carbs, it's important to look at how you eat those carbs because eating carbs on their own can lead to quick spikes in both blood sugar and insulin, which will interrupt your fat loss. Instead, you should pair each carb you eat with protein and fat sources.

When you add proteins and fats to your carbs, it slows down your digestion, so glucose is released more gradually into your bloodstream than if you eat the carbs on their own. Eating proteins and fats with your carbs keeps your blood sugar levels lower, and it also helps you feel full longer, which reduces your risk of overeating.

For example, if you're having a slice of fruit, think about pairing it with a few nuts to increase the fat content. Or if you're having a slice of bread, make sure you pair it with something high fat, such as an avocado. This small change in how you eat carbs changes how both blood sugar and insulin is spiked in your body, and therefore it helps both your weight-loss efforts and your metabolic health!

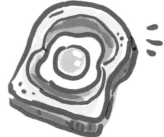

FOOD ORDER MATTERS

How you order the foods during your meal also affects your blood sugar and insulin response. Research has found that eating carbs at the end of your meal, after having your proteins and fats, can reduce the insulin spike they cause.[2]

Eating this way lets your body start to process proteins and fats first, which prepares your body to handle the glucose from carbs more efficiently.

Using the strategy of food order is a really simple and powerful way to hack your metabolism. I recommend that you start your meal with high-fat protein and fats and then move on to low-carb carbohydrates toward the end of your meal. Aside from controlling your blood sugar levels, eating this way makes you feel fuller, which prevents you from eating too much and overindulging in high-carb foods. I love this hack because changing the order in which you eat the different components of your meal is so simple, and you get great benefit without actually changing the ingredients of what you're eating.

USING FIBER and ACID to SUPERCHARGE YOUR WEIGHT LOSS

Adding fiber and acid to your diet is another simple way to lose some extra weight because they change how carbs are processed and absorbed in your body.

Fiber makes you feel fuller, slows down how quickly carbs are absorbed by your body, and helps you have a healthier gut microbiome—all things that can help you lose more weight. You can find fiber in low-carb vegetables such as broccoli and cauliflower, but you can also add fiber to your diet by taking a fiber supplement such as psyllium husk.

Acid, such as from lemon juice or apple cider vinegar, is great for your gut microbiome. When you add something acidic to your meals (or have a bit of lemon juice or apple cider vinegar before your meals), you reduce the glycemic impact of the foods you're eating. The acid lowers both your blood sugar and your insulin levels,[3] which helps you lose weight and improves your insulin sensitivity.

It's super easy to add fiber and acid to your diet. Start each meal with a shot of lemon juice or apple cider vinegar mixed with water, and take a fiber supplement half an hour before you eat. Another option is to add a lemon vinaigrette to your salads and eat plenty of low-carb vegetables.

Making these simple adjustments to your diet changes how your body responds to carbs to help you lose more weight with very little extra effort. Win-win!

FERMENTED FOODS and YOUR GUT MICROBIOME

Frequently eating fermented foods can contribute to a healthier gut microbiome, and having a healthy gut microbiome supports not only your digestion but also has a positive impact on your insulin resistance, immune system, mood, and mental health.

When you have fermented foods and drinks like yogurt, kimchi, sauerkraut, apple cider vinegar, and kombucha, it helps you actively diversify your gut bacteria, which is important for your overall health.

There has recently been more research into how fermented foods can modify your gut microbiome,[4] and studies show that eating fermented foods can lead to lower inflammatory markers in the body. One study found that people who consume fermented foods reduce several inflammatory compounds, including those associated with type 2 diabetes and rheumatoid arthritis. People who consume fermented foods were also found to have a more diverse array of microbes in their gut.[5] Having a diverse gut microbiome is incredibly beneficial, but people often lack this diversity because highly processed diets and modern ways of eating and living don't promote it.

You can easily add fermented foods into your diet to encourage diversity in your gut microbiome. Add sauerkraut or kimchi as a side dish to meals you're already planning to eat, mix apple cider vinegar in water to drink before your meal, or have full-fat yogurt with a handful of strawberries or coconut chips as a keto dessert.

SWEETENERS and WHY THEY STALL WEIGHT LOSS

As you know, consuming high levels of sugar spikes your blood sugar and insulin levels, and those spikes promote fat storage and weight gain and increase your chances of developing type 2 diabetes. Sweeteners have therefore been viewed as a "healthier alternative" because they don't spike blood sugar.

You might be tempted to use artificial or natural sweeteners as a sugar substitute so you can keep enjoying desserts or other sweet things without the high calories or insulin spikes of sugar.

However, blood sugar is just one piece of the puzzle, and although blood sugar and insulin are related, they are not the same thing. The fact that sweeteners don't affect blood sugar levels doesn't mean they don't have an effect on your insulin levels.

Some studies have shown that although sweeteners don't spike blood sugar, they can actually spike insulin.[6] Other studies have shown that consuming sweeteners not only causes an insulin spike but also increases insulin resistance,[7] and both of these facts are crucial knowledge if you're trying to lose body fat.

Insulin is a fat-storage hormone, so when insulin levels are high, your body stores body fat. When insulin levels are low, your body burns body fat. Blood sugar is a measure of the amount of sugar present in your blood at a given time, which means that even if a sweetener doesn't spike blood sugar (because it isn't sugar), if it spikes insulin levels, it still leads to fat storage.

The reason sweeteners can spike insulin without spiking blood sugar is because you're essentially tricking your body to expect sugar. When you eat or drink something with sweeteners, your body will think it's getting sugar because sweeteners taste sweet. Tricking your body in this way results in your body overcompensating by increasing your cravings and appetite and releasing more insulin but not processing it properly, which eventually leads to insulin resistance.[8] Of course, having an increased appetite will only make fasting much more difficult than it has to be.

It can be difficult to understand and measure how sweeteners affect your body. Many people regularly check their blood sugar levels at home using a glucose monitor to see how different foods affect their blood sugar, which helps them make better choices about their diet. I frequently hear people say, "I drink Diet Coke or take sweeteners in my coffee, and it doesn't affect my insulin." But these people are actually talking about their *blood sugar levels*, not their *insulin levels*, and are confused about the difference.

Measuring insulin levels is a complicated process and can only be done at a lab, so it's not something that just anybody can measure at home on a daily basis. Because of this difference, a lot of people consume sweeteners and think they're making a healthier choice because of their low blood sugar readings, but they're unaware of the insulin spikes that could be stalling or otherwise negatively affecting their weight loss.

I see this with clients all the time. When one of my clients experiences a weight-loss stall, I always ask if they've had any sweeteners. That's when the truth comes out. They've either been drinking some flavored water or taking sweeteners in their coffee. I immediately tell them to stop, and, begrudgingly, they do. Lo and behold, as soon as they stop the sweeteners, their weight starts moving again.

It's incredibly important to understand the relationship between sweeteners and insulin levels when you're fasting. Because sweeteners can impact insulin levels, they aren't safe to be consumed while fasting because anything that spikes insulin breaks your fast. So contrary to what a lot of people tell you, zero-calorie drinks, including diet sodas or anything else with sweeteners, aren't "safe" to consume during a fast.

And while a lot of people say they've had diet drinks and still lost weight on a fast, it's important to note that losing weight does not necessarily mean you're *fasting*. You can lose weight in a variety of ways, including extreme caloric restriction, but that doesn't mean you're *fasting*. You can lose weight by eating only salads several times a day, but eating salads doesn't mean you're *fasting*. And the same goes for drinking zero-calorie drinks. Although you can lose weight while consuming sweeteners, it doesn't mean you're *fasting*, and it may stall or slow your weight loss. My recommendation is that you always to stay clear of zero-calorie drinks or anything else containing sweeteners, artificial flavorings, or natural flavorings while fasting because any of these things may spike your insulin and break your fast.

In the next chapter, I talk about the ketogenic diet and how to do it correctly to maximize both your health and weight-loss benefits.

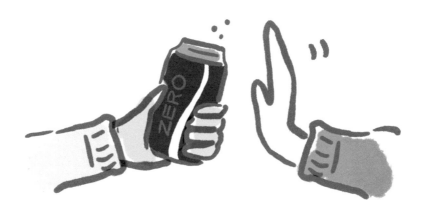

CHAPTER 13
THE KETO DIET

The ketogenic (keto) diet focuses on eating high fat, moderate protein, and low carbs to force your body into ketosis. In other words, both fasting and the keto diet work to achieve the same thing: They trigger your body to switch from using carbs for fuel to burning your stored body fat for fuel.

When you're fasting, you're naturally putting your body into ketosis as your body uses up its glucose stores. When you eat a ketogenic diet during your eating window, you're staying in ketosis even when you're not fasting. So when you pair intermittent fasting with eating a keto diet, you can speed up ketosis and boost the benefits of fasting.

In this chapter, I walk you through how to incorporate the keto diet into your fasting lifestyle.

HOW to DO KETO CORRECTLY

To follow the keto diet correctly and get your body to stay in ketosis even when you're eating, you need to limit your carbs to less than 20 grams of net carbs per day. You can do so easily by cutting all bread, pasta, sugar, flour, rice, legumes, and fruit from your diet. Instead, you eat fatty cuts of meat, green above-ground vegetables, unprocessed oils (such as olive oil and coconut oil), and animal fats such as butter, lard, and heavy cream. Be careful about eating too much protein because excess protein can turn into glucose through a process called gluconeogenesis, which can disrupt ketosis.

But as long as you stick to these three food groups and make sure to eat only until you're satisfied, there's usually no need to weigh your ingredients and track macros. Some people find it helpful to track carbs for the first couple of weeks to get a good idea of what 20 grams of carbs actually looks like. To stay safely in ketosis, aim to consume 0.5 to 0.9 gram of protein per pound of your target weight. These amounts will ensure that your body is getting enough protein to support muscle maintenance without

weight gain. Getting kicked out of ketosis by eating too much protein is uncommon, but you can make sure that you're on track by checking for signs of ketosis, such as feeling less hungry or having a metallic taste in your mouth, which is known as "keto breath."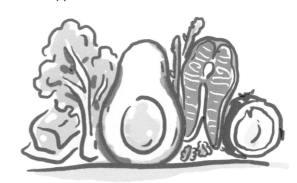

HOW LOW-CARB VERSUS HIGH-CARB FOODS AFFECT YOUR INSULIN

The keto diet limits the amount of carbs you eat, which changes how insulin is released in your body.

High-carb foods spike your blood sugar and insulin, which tells your body to store energy as fat. On the other hand, when you cut the carbs, you cut the fat storage. Eating a keto diet keeps your blood sugar low, which leads to less insulin being released, and your body receives the message to burn fat instead of storing it. This makes you lose weight, reduces your insulin resistance, and improves your insulin sensitivity—all of which help protect you from developing type 2 diabetes and other metabolic issues.

WHAT YOU CAN EAT on a KETO DIET

To keep your body in ketosis, you need to be selective about what you eat. Here, I provide a simple list of foods that you can eat on a keto diet:

Pick a PROTEIN	Pick a VEGGIE (or 2)	Add FAT
• Chicken	• Cauliflower	• Butter
• Steak	• Brocolli	• Oil
• Fish	• Squash	• Lard
• Pork	• Zuchinni	• Ghee
• Ground beef	• Asparagus	• Cheese
• Turkey	• Brussel sprouts	• Bacon
• Lamb	• Salad	• Avocado
• Venison	• Radish	• Pork rinds
• Seafood	• Jicama	• Eggs
• Eggs	• Green beans	
	• Green pepper	
	• Cucumber	
	• Onion	

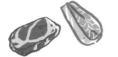

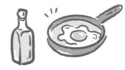

Following a keto diet isn't only about the foods you eat. It's also about the foods you avoid. Foods you should stay away from include these:

- Sugar
- Flour
- Grains
- Rice
- Fruits
- Legumes
- Root vegetables
- Low-fat and diet products

WHY FAKE KETO FOODS SABOTAGE YOUR WEIGHT-LOSS EFFORTS

When you're on a keto diet, you will inevitably come across a bunch of highly processed, supposedly "keto-friendly" foods on the supermarket shelves. I always recommend that you stay away from these so-called keto products. I call them Frankenfoods because they're not really food.

They're highly processed, commercially sold products (for example, keto brownies, keto bread, and keto ice cream) posing as keto-friendly foods, but they're actually not keto at all. In actual fact, these Frankenfoods not only stall your weight loss but also take you away from the very core of the ketogenic diet—which is to clean up what you eat.

The reason these types of foods are so sneaky is that the companies behind them use marketing tactics to make it seem like they're keto when they actually aren't. A lot of these foods display their carb content per serving size to make the carb content look low. Doing it this way allows companies to make foods that aren't keto seem keto friendly to the untrained eye. The truth is that the serving sizes of foods like these are usually quite small—probably smaller than what you'd consider a serving—and if you make a serving small enough, any food can be made "keto."

What you really need to look at is not the carb content per serving but the carb content per 100 grams. When you look at carbs per 100 grams, you're able to get a more accurate carb content reading, and you'll have a much easier time determining which foods are actually keto and which are not. A lot of American food labels don't display carbs per 100 grams as standard, so you might have to bring out your calculator for this. *As a general rule, you should aim for the majority of your keto foods and ingredients to have less than 5 to 7 grams of carbs per 100 grams.*

Use these steps to calculate carbs per 100 grams from the information on a US nutrition label:

1. Find the serving size. All nutrition labels display a "per serving" calculation and indicate how many grams a suggested serving is. I'm using some keto brownies as an example, and one serving is 24 grams ($\frac{1}{12}$ brownie).

2. Find the number of net carbs per serving by subtracting the fiber and sugar alcohol (sweeteners) content from the total carbs—in this case 17 minus 4 minus 5. The net carbs per serving is 8 grams.

3. Divide the net carbs by the serving size (24) to get the number of carbs per gram. 8/24 = 0.33.

4. Multiply this by 100 to get the net carbs per 100 grams = 33 grams.

European nutrition labels are usually much easier to decipher because they tend to already have a separate section for nutrition content per 100 grams. Also, fiber and sugar alcohols are already subtracted from the carb count. So all you have to do is look at the "carbs per 100 grams" section to find the correct value.

Note: If the food item contains sweeteners, they're listed as "sugar alcohols," and you subtract these from the carbs per 100 grams to calculate the net carbs.

It doesn't stop there, though. Not only are the carb counts misleading, but processed keto foods usually contain a bunch of additives, sweeteners, and preservatives that can disrupt your gut health and lead to higher inflammation in your body.

Instead of buying these highly processed, commercially packaged foods, stick to whole, single-ingredient foods—items that aren't processed and contain no added sugars, fillers, or complicated ingredients. Always look for foods that exist in their natural state and have just one ingredient, such as pieces of meat, fish, and chicken that aren't processed. The same goes for vegetables; pick raw vegetables from the fresh produce aisle, like broccoli, cauliflower, asparagus, and cucumber. Single-ingredient foods like these provide your body with essential nutrients without unnecessary carbs or other additives found in processed, boxed, and ready-made foods.

The more you rely on highly processed and convenient foods, the more you're getting away from developing the healthier eating habits that will ensure you're successful on your weight-loss journey in the long run. So if something comes from a box, a bag, or a packet and sounds too good to be true, it most likely is.

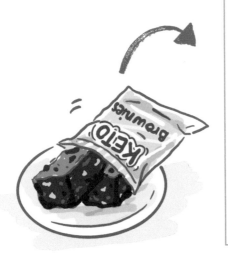

NUTRITION FACTS

Serving size: 24 g
Serving per container: 12

	Per Serving Per 1/12 baked brownie		Carbs Per 100 g
Calories	200		833
	%DV*		
Total Fat	13 g	17%	54 g
Saturated Fat	5 g	25%	20 g
Trans Fat	0 g		0 g
Cholesterol	45 mg	15%	187 mg
Sodium	115 mg	5%	479 mg
Total Carb	17 g	6%	70 g
Dietary Fiber	4 g	4%	16 g
Total Sugars	<1 g	x	4 g
Incl. Added Sugars	0 g	0%	0 g
Sugar Alcohol	5 g		20 g
Protein	3 g		12 g

Carbs per serving:
17-4-5-8 g

looks keto...

Carbs per 100 g:
70-16-20-34 g

...but isn't keto

HOW to EAT KETO at RESTAURANTS

At some point, you'll need to have a meal at a restaurant. You might think that sticking to your keto diet in these situations is impossible because carbs are everywhere, but you're wrong. Eating keto at restaurants is actually one of the easiest and most straightforward things you can do.

Finding keto options at restaurants doesn't have to be complicated! The key is to make it as easy as possible for yourself. Start by looking up the restaurant's menu online before you go. This way you can pick out keto-friendly meals ahead of time to help you avoid being overwhelmed when you get there. Feeling overwhelmed increases the likelihood that you'll be tempted to go off track.

The first thing you should start with is picking a meat. Almost all restaurants, whether it's a steakhouse, a seafood restaurant, or your local diner or takeaway joint, will have some type of fish, beef, pork, or chicken. Pick an option that's not battered or breaded or covered in sauce. Batters, breadings, and sauces aren't keto.

The second thing you want to do is to swap out the side. Carby sides are usually standard accompaniments, but most restaurants will let you swap the side for either steamed or grilled vegetables. You also can order a side salad and have your meat with that. Don't be afraid to ask for substitutions. Most restaurants are used to dietary requirements and allergies and have no problem swapping out their sides if you ask them to.

Many sauces and stews are high in sugar and have been thickened with flour or cornstarch, so they are not keto friendly. Stay away from them. As long as your meat is prepared on its own without being covered in sauce, you'll most likely be fine.

If you choose to have a salad, be very careful about the dressing. Most dressings are full of sugar and are definitely not keto. You can have a salad, but order it without the dressing or ask for olive oil, lemon juice, or vinegar on the side. This way you can make sure your salad is keto friendly.

HOW to MANAGE YOUR AT-HOME MEALS: KEEP IT BORING

When you swap to a completely new way of eating, it can be overwhelming and confusing. When there are many new things to think about, you want to keep things as simple as possible. This is why I always recommend keeping your food menu as "boring" as possible. The point is not to take away the joy of eating or force yourself to eat things you don't like. The goal is to streamline your diet and your food choices to make eating as manageable and sustainable as possible.

Here are some benefits of a "boring" menu:

- **Reduced decision fatigue:** When you have a set menu of meals to choose from every day, your mental load is decreased because you have fewer decisions to make about your diet, which frees up your mental energy for other things.

- **Simpler grocery shopping:** When you know exactly which ingredients you need for your "boring" meals, shopping becomes a lot more straightforward, which saves you time and energy and prevents you from straying down the middle aisles.

- **Easier macro tracking:** I don't usually track macros, and certainly not calories, but when you're just starting out with the keto diet, it can be helpful to track your macros for a couple of weeks so you know what 20 grams of carbs looks like. Eating the same meals every day makes tracking so much simpler.

- **Consistency leads to success**: A consistent diet is easier to follow, and we all know that consistency is what leads to sustainable weight loss in the long run.

The concept of "boring" meals is really straightforward: Pick a few meals that you like and then rotate through them regularly. (You might find some new favorites among the recipes in Part 3 of this book.) When you're building your menu, remember to focus on single-ingredient foods that you enjoy. Stay away from highly processed things—foods that come in a box, bag, or packet.

It's important to choose ingredients and meals that you actually like because it helps you to stick to your routine without feeling deprived. Some of my favorite meals include smoked salmon and scrambled eggs, steak with broccoli, and chicken with sautéed garlic mushrooms and asparagus. These meals are keto friendly, and they give me a good balance of simplicity and nutrition. They have very few ingredients and require little preparation, but they're delicious and filling, I look forward to eating them.

Having a "boring" food menu doesn't mean you have to sacrifice on flavor or enjoyment. While the base of your menu may be simple or basic, I always recommend that you experiment with different spices and herbs, add plenty of butter or olive oil, and swap out your vegetables and proteins frequently to keep your meals fresh and interesting. The less you have to think about your food each day, the easier this journey will be for you.

CLIENT SPOTLIGHT: ANNALIESE

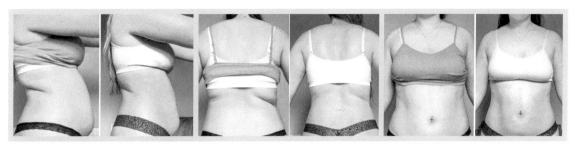

STARTING WEIGHT	**180 lbs**
CURRENT WEIGHT	**145 lbs**
TOTAL WEIGHT LOST	**35 lbs**

I am going to start from the very beginning of my weight struggles, which was the dreaded COVID-19 pandemic. I know I'm not the only person who went into lockdown and found the only thing to do was to watch movies and eat.

I had always worn a UK size 8 (a US size 4). I didn't realize how much weight I was gaining because I was lounging around in comfy clothes all the time. Eventually when the restrictions started to lift, I tried a pair of my favorite jeans, and I struggled to get them over my thighs. I thought maybe I'd only gone up a size. Then I started trying on new clothes and realized I'd gone up three sizes. I was now a UK size 14 (US size 10) and 180 pounds. This may not seem bad to a lot of people, but as someone who had never been over a size 8, this was a drastic change for me. I became very self-conscious. I lived in tracksuits so nobody could see how much weight I'd put on. I had red stretch marks everywhere, even on my arms, and my skin was breaking out horribly as well!

This was the breaking point for me, and I knew I wanted to lose some weight so I could feel confident enough to wear the clothes I wanted to wear again. I spent around six months trying to calorie count and put myself into calorie deficits, going to the gym, and getting more steps in every day. None of those things did much for me. I thought maybe I was doing too much or too little of a deficit, so I sought professional help from a personal trainer and did group training sessions twice a week for six weeks. I ate the meals the personal trainer prepared for me, and at the end of the six weeks, I had lost only 2 pounds. The rest of the group had lost a good bit more than I had, and even the personal trainer didn't understand why I hadn't lost more. I was doing everything right! I felt so defeated because of the amount of work I was putting into losing weight and nothing was coming from it. I started snacking a lot again, and I gave up completely.

A few months later, I was scrolling on TikTok and saw one of Emma's videos on fasting. The video explained how it worked and showed results. I was skeptical at first, as anyone would be. After this video, I started doing my own research to see if this was something I wanted to try. After feeling defeated twice already, I feared the same situation would happen again. However, if you don't try, you'll never know.

When I started fasting with Emma's help, I mainly stuck to twenty-four- to forty-eight-hour fasts with low-carb meals. Within the first week of fasting, I lost 7 pounds! I was elated! I couldn't believe this had happened so fast, and it wasn't difficult at all. I just kept my steps up every day and drank 2 to 3 liters of water a day, which also helped my skin a lot. This result motivated me more, and I couldn't wait to see how much more I could lose. Fast-forward to a month of fasting: I had lost a total of 21 pounds! I went from 180 pounds to 159 pounds, and I lost inches everywhere. I was down to a size 12 by this point.

My birthday came, and I wore a tight dress and felt more confident than I had in years. My original plan had been to lose weight for my birthday. But I loved fasting so much because it made my body feel great, my skin health better, my hair stronger and shinier, and my energy levels throughout the day better, so I decided to continue with fasting to lose some more weight before my holiday, which was four months after my birthday. My new goal was to get down to 145 pounds by the time my vacation came. I thought it was a bit optimistic but not an unachievable goal. Soon after this, I hit a fasting plateau, and I freaked out that I couldn't lose any more weight. I switched up my fasting routine from twenty-four hours to forty-eight hours, and I ended up hitting my goal weight two-and-a-half months later.

It's almost been a year from when I started my journey with fasting, and I have kept the weight off. I only fast now and again. I still eat takeaways and chocolate. In fact, I never restricted myself from these treats, which is why I found fasting to be maintainable. I will always recommend fasting to anyone who wants to feel better about themselves. People always ask me if it's worth it, and my response is always yes. Feeling better about myself was worth it to me, and the other benefits that came along with it were a great bonus.

CHAPTER 14
MINDFUL EATING AND MAINTENANCE

One of the biggest challenges to weight loss and maintenance relates to food mindset. It's something I work on with my clients every day.

Using mindful eating with fasting helped me reach my goal weight and is one of the things I use to maintain my weight as well. *Mindful eating* simply means tuning in to your body's needs and cues regarding how it feels when you eat and drink to guide you to make balanced and emotionally healthy food choices.

The idea behind mindful eating is that when you regularly check in with yourself, you reduce your risk of overeating or mindlessly munching for reasons other than hunger (for example, emotional eating or comfort eating). One of the main aims of mindful eating is to help you achieve food freedom, which is no longer letting food control or overwhelm you. Because of mindful eating, I learned to be calmer around food.

Mindful eating is connected to the concept of *intuitive eating*, which involves learning to listen to your body regarding what food it needs without guilt or shame.[1] But intuitive eating is often misunderstood and misused. A lot of people see it as an excuse to overindulge in empty-calorie foods, but this isn't true. Intuitive eating isn't simply "eat whatever you want, whenever you want"—that's *impulsive eating*. The first part of mindful eating and achieving food freedom is having the *freedom to say yes* to all the foods you want to have. But it's important not to forget about the second part of the equation: having the *freedom to say no* to foods when you're not hungry or when food isn't what your body or mind needs at that time.

Many of us have become so disconnected from our natural hunger and fullness cues that we no longer eat only when we're truly hungry. Instead, we eat for a number of other reasons including habit, because we're told to eat, for convenience, or just because food is put in front of us. How many times have you had a slice of dry, unsatisfying cake at the office simply because it was there? Or sat down for lunch just because it was lunchtime? Having a busy schedule coupled with eating highly processed, high-carb, and high-sugar foods wreak havoc on your hormones and make it difficult for you to be in tune with your body. Because people so disconnected from their natural cues, many rely on fad diets that artificially limit how much or what they eat to try (and ultimately fail) to reach their weight-loss goals. You've probably gone on a restrictive diet many times only to give up and proceed to shovel everything into your mouth after just a couple of weeks. This constant cycle of restriction and overeating causes weight gain, emotional eating, and a negative relationship with food. For you to achieve and maintain your goal weight, you need to find calm and balance around food, and mindful eating is the way to do that.

REASONS to PRACTICE MINDFUL EATING

Mindful eating isn't easy, but with practice it can change how you relate to food and your body. The goal is to achieve food freedom and food neutrality, where you can enjoy a wide variety of foods without feeling deprived or restricted, and you see foods as neither "good" nor "bad."

But again, mindful eating is not a free-for-all or an excuse to overindulge in highly processed foods. Only eat what you truly need, and learn to listen to your body's cues. This also means that you need to consider your past experiences with eating certain types of foods and how they make you feel. If a big bowl of pasta or a whole box of doughnuts is what you crave, but eating that food would make you feel horrible and nauseated afterward, not eating it is what you need.

Again, this is the difference between mindful eating and impulsive eating. A craving for a food is only part of the equation; it doesn't automatically mean you have to eat it. Don't eat just because you have a craving or just because food is offered. Use all the available data. Are you actually hungry? Or are you sad? Stressed? Emotional? Bored? Will eating this food make you feel good and satisfied in your body and mind? By understanding the difference between emotional hunger and physical hunger, between eating for nourishment and eating for comfort, you can start to make choices that create balance in your body *and* mind.

MINDFUL EATING TECHNIQUES

There are a few different ways you can practice mindful eating.

The first one is to take small bites and chew each bite carefully. One of my favorite ways to do so is to put my knife and fork down between each bite. I only pick them up once I've finished a bite and feel ready for the next. Chew each bite carefully, and make sure you taste the flavors and textures of each bite. Ask yourself how the food feels in your mouth. Is it crunchy, soft, or creamy? What flavors are coming through? Is it salty, sweet, or bitter? And what other sensations do you feel? Is the food hot or cold? Tuning in with each bite in this way keeps you engaged so that you're paying full attention to what you're doing—which leads to my second point around mindful leading: Never eat when you're distracted.

If you're watching TV, scrolling your phone, or driving while you're eating, you will easily munch away mindlessly and end up eating more than you intend. To practice mindful eating successfully, you should turn your tech off and not occupy yourself with any other distractions during this time. This includes TV, cell phone, podcasts, or reading. Spending time with yourself and food "alone" in this way can feel challenging in the beginning, but it teaches you how to eat in a calm and healthy way.

Next, you want to make sure that you tune in carefully to your hunger and fullness cues. It can take up to twenty minutes of eating before your body registers that you're full. So make sure that you eat at a comfortable pace, and keep checking in with yourself about how you're feeling. After each bite, ask yourself if you're still hungry. If you're not still hungry, you have the sign that you're satisfied and you've had enough. People often eat to the point of absolute fullness, but this is actually eating too much. You're better off stopping where you have a more neutral and comfortable feeling.

If you're not used to eating in this way, it can take a little while to get used to. Eating only until you're satisfied is quite a neutral feeling; it's the point where you're just not hungry anymore. As soon as you sense that you're satisfied, push your plate to the side and end your meal. It doesn't matter if there's more food on your plate at that point. Your body has told you that it's done. So either save the remaining food for later or throw it away. Don't finish food on your plate if you've reached the point of satisfaction.

The same goes for listening to your hunger cues. As you've learned, hunger comes and goes in waves, and sometimes it's appropriate to listen to that hunger. Other times, it's not. For example, if you're in the middle of a planned fast and you feel hungry, it's perfectly OK to ignore that feeling for a while until it's time to eat. Hunger during your fasting window is not a cause for alarm. It's a normal response in the body that naturally passes without you needing to do anything about it.

You should also never eat if you're not hungry. If you reach your eating window, but you're not hungry, don't eat. You're better off waiting until your body tells you that it's ready for food rather than forcing yourself to eat when you're not hungry. Your body is learning how to use stored body fat for energy, and it's important that you let it do that.

FOOD NEUTRALITY and FINDING FOOD FREEDOM

Another important part of mindful eating is removing your emotional attachment and triggers to food, with the ultimate goal of achieving food neutrality.

Food neutrality just means that you don't see any food as inherently "good" or "bad." Labeling foods as good or bad can make your cravings worse, so try to have a more neutral attitude around food.

The ultimate goal of mindful eating is for you to develop food freedom. This is where you can be completely free around food, and you don't have any fears about certain foods triggering you or causing you to binge. Achieving food freedom means you can have all the processed and high-carb foods in your home without being tempted to eat them because they're not what you're eating right now. Food freedom means moving away from thinking, "I *can't* have that," and instead thinking, "I *choose* not to have that because it's not what my body and mind needs right now." By giving yourself *permission* to eat whatever foods you like but at the same time giving yourself agency to decide not to have them if they don't serve you, you can start to remove the power that certain foods hold over you.

Mindful eating is all about taking back your power and not letting yourself be controlled by food. When you have this perspective, it helps you reduce your guilt and anxiety about eating, and it helps you develop a more balanced approach to food.

Developing food neutrality and food freedom is so important because emotional eating can completely throw off both your weight loss and your maintenance plan. Mindful eating can help you find the emotional triggers behind your eating. Once you know your triggers, you can find other ways to deal with your stress, boredom, and other feelings instead of turning to food. For example, you can pick up a hobby, talk to a friend, go for a walk, or use relaxation techniques like yoga or meditation.

FASTING and MINDFUL EATING

Fasting can be a powerful tool for mindful eating. When you fast, you give your body a break from food and allow it to burn its stored fat for energy.

It also gives you plenty of time to think about how your cravings affect you and use stress-reducing activities such as mindfulness and meditation instead of giving in to your cravings.

On top of that, fasting, especially when paired with a ketogenic diet, helps reset your body's hormone levels, which reduces both your cravings and hunger.[2] By fasting, you reset your unhealthy food cravings, which makes you better able to tune in to your body's true hunger and fullness cues. Combining fasting with mindful eating will help you maintain your weight loss in the long run.

PATIENCE

Many times, mindful eating might not work right away. Because you've spent years eating high-carb and high-sugar foods, you've most likely dysregulated your hormones and metabolism so much that you crave these highly processed foods all the time.

That's why using fasting along with a ketogenic diet to heal your metabolic profile first is so important. After that, you can use mindful eating to develop a sustainable way of eating and living that will help you achieve food freedom and maintain your weight for the rest of your life.

The key is to be patient enough to take it slow and keep practicing until it becomes a natural part of how you eat. Incorporating mindful eating into your fasting journey helps you develop a healthy mindset around food. Through this process, you can make peace with food and find a balanced way to maintain your weight loss in the long run.

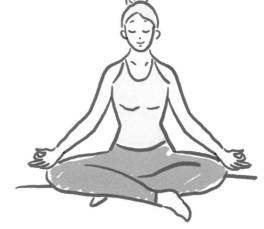

RAIN: An ACRONYM for MINDFUL EATING

A great tool for overcoming emotional eating, mindless eating, or overeating involves pausing before you act on a thought or impulse. RAIN is an acronym coined by Buddhist teacher Michele McDonald and adapted by Tara Brach that can help immensely when you're tempted to eat mindlessly or give into emotional eating. The illustration shows what RAIN stands for.

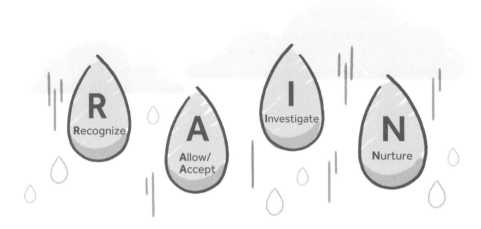

The first step is to recognize when you're tempted to eat emotionally. Often, you don't even realize you're in automatic eating mode until much later. This step is all about *recognizing* the temptation to eat emotionally or overeat before *acting* on it. This way you can catch yourself in the act and acknowledge when you're experiencing a craving that isn't driven by true hunger. This initial recognition, or stopping in your tracks, is often the first key to breaking the cycle of emotional eating. By being aware of your thoughts and feelings in those moments, you can begin to take back control and not give in to unhealthy coping patterns.

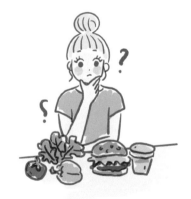

The second step is to allow or accept that you want to eat emotionally or mindlessly. It's about accepting that you have a craving or desire to eat emotionally and letting that feeling sit with you without acting on it. This way, you can give yourself permission to experience the craving without judgment or guilt. It's important to know that the feeling or craving itself isn't going to harm you or do anything to you, and it's OK to have those thoughts. Simply having a thought or craving doesn't mean you've failed. Don't push the feeling away or judge yourself for having it. Simply sit with it, observe it, and let it be there. No one can make you act on a feeling or craving other than you. By accepting that the feeling or craving exists and calmly allowing yourself to feel it and observe it without fear, you can start to develop a calmer and healthier approach to food decisions.

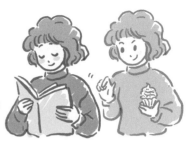

Third, you need to investigate why you're having the craving or impulse to eat emotionally in the first place. Are you truly hungry for that food? Or are you bored? Sad? Lonely? Anxious? Perhaps you want to procrastinate to avoid work or chores you know need to be done. Whatever the reason, get curious and narrow down the origin of the feeling. Then ask yourself if you can alleviate that feeling without turning to food.

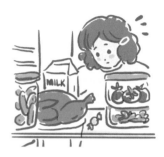

The final step, nurture, is about showing yourself grace and compassion and recognizing that almost everyone struggles with emotional or mindless eating at some point. Struggling with, or even giving in to, emotional eating doesn't make you a bad person, and it doesn't reflect poorly on your character or willpower. It's simply something that happens to certain people in response to certain triggers at certain times. Forgive yourself and then quickly move on. By approaching yourself with love and compassion, you can start to break free from the guilt and shame cycle that usually brings people right back to emotional eating all over again.

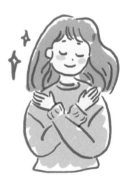

After following the steps in this acronym, you decide how to proceed. This process itself won't stop you from diving headfirst into the snack box. *You* have the ultimate power to choose what you do or don't do in response to any situation. But going through the RAIN thought process allows you to slow down and reflect on the decisions you're about to make, hit the pause button, and get in touch with your intuition.

MAINTENANCE: WHAT'S NEXT AFTER REACHING YOUR WEIGHT-LOSS GOAL?

When you've used all my methods and tips and tricks and finally achieved your weight-loss goal, how do you make sure that you maintain it?

Maintenance is a completely different beast than the weight-loss phase, and I struggled quite a lot with this part. The techniques and habits you lean on in maintenance are not necessarily the same as the ones you used to lose your weight, so it might take some time to figure out. My journey to maintenance wasn't straightforward. I struggled a bit with weight gain in the beginning because I didn't know how to strike a good balance between fasting and eating. But ever since I cracked the code to maintenance, I've been able to maintain my weight for years. In this section, I share my favorite tips for maintenance success.

Intermittent Fasting for Maintenance

One of my biggest tips for maintenance is to still include some form of intermittent fasting in your routine, but you don't have to do it as frequently as you did when you were losing weight. Intermittent fasting is great for weight loss, but it's also incredibly useful for maintaining the results once you've achieved them. Since you're done with losing weight, you can't use the same fasting schedule to maintain your weight, or you'll risk losing even more weight. So you need to do some tweaking to find what works for you.

When you're in maintenance, you can be a bit more flexible with your fasting. For example, you might follow a 16:8 schedule to maintain your weight on most days, but you might want to take Saturdays and Sundays off to eat breakfast or brunch with your family. Or you might want to use a method where you eat normally for five days and do one-meal-a day (OMAD) on two days.

Maintenance looks different for everyone, so you might need some time to figure it out. You'll want to find a sweet spot that enables you to maintain your weight without losing more or regaining the weight that you lost. The beauty with maintenance is that you can be a lot more flexible than when you were in your weight-loss phase. Once your goal weight is stable, you can usually have a few days when you're not fasting at all without any great consequences.

Reintroducing Carbs

One of the most common questions I'm asked is whether I still cut carbs now that I'm in maintenance. And the answer is no. While I still try to be mindful about my consumption of highly processed carbs, I've slowly reintroduced carbohydrates into my diet, and I don't follow a strict keto diet in maintenance. That being said, a lot of people successfully follow a ketogenic diet in maintenance because they find that that's what makes them feel the best. Again, maintenance is different for everyone, so it's up to you to find what works for you.

If you decide that you want to reintroduce carbs, it's important that you choose the right types of carbs. Make sure you focus on whole, single-ingredient foods, like fruits and vegetables, not processed carbs out of a box or packet. I highly recommend that you avoid processed carbs because they cause bigger insulin spikes and will undo all the hard work you've gone through to heal your metabolic and gut health through fasting and a low-carb diet. Remember: Carbs don't have to equal a crappy, highly processed diet. Vegetables are carbs too.

Reintroducing carbs can be tricky business, and different types of carbs cause different types of responses in your body. Make sure you give yourself some time to experiment with trial and error to see which types of foods your body reacts the best to.

And always make sure you eat fiber and acid before any serving of carbs because they reduce the carbs' impact on your insulin levels.

Finding What Works for You

The true key to maintenance is finding what works for you. As I've said, maintenance looks different for everyone, so what works for others might not work for you, and vice versa.

Try finding a way of life that you're comfortable following whether, it's a Monday, a Saturday, or a vacation day. If you ever find yourself straying from your idea of a balanced and healthy diet, simply make sure you get back on track without overcompensating, or you'll risk ending up in a binge-and-restrict cycle.

Make sure you keep following the principles of never eating if you're not hungry, always stop eating when you're satisfied, and never use food as an emotional crutch.

CLIENT SPOTLIGHT: CARLY

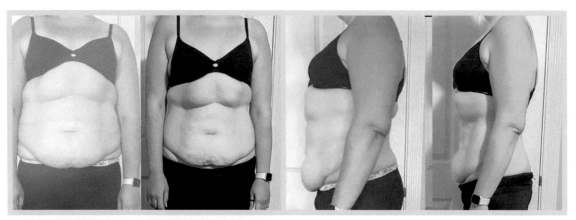

STARTING WEIGHT	**265 lbs**
CURRENT WEIGHT	**205 lbs**
TOTAL WEIGHT LOST	**60 lbs**

When I was around 7 years old, I started coming home from school with anxiety, and my mom would always greet me at the door with a sweet treat. As I grew older, I found that the only reaction I had to any stress whatsoever was to eat. The quick hit of dopamine was what got me through the years of bullying and general teenage drama, and I grew to be "the fat kid" in my school. Once I got out of school, I developed an even unhealthier relationship with food because I was now able to use my own money to explore even greasier and sweeter options, and my weight and health spiraled out of control. I would binge eat, purge, and exercise until I threw up, and I would try every yo-yo fad diet that I could possibly try. I am 180 cm (5'11") tall, and the heaviest I ever got was 300 pounds. I loved exercise, but I would do it only to burn calories. I loved going out with friends, but I always had to check the menu for what calories were in each option. I was living my life, but I was miserable thinking about how I would work off the next meal. And if I didn't see a weight drop on the scale, it would send me into another 4,500-calorie binge in one sitting. I felt heavy and sluggish, and I had so much heartburn. My legs ached all the time. I was ready to just let the food demon inside of me win and take me to my new 600-pound life.

I was introduced to the idea of fasting for my health a couple years ago when I opened up a keto bakery. I love the psychology behind fasting; I could take control of when I eat. The first time I fasted, I remember craving only healthy foods. Instead of constantly wanting sweets and overly refined treats, I was craving the crunch of celery and the rich flavor of a nicely cooked steak. I suddenly felt physically lighter, and it made the mental battle that I had always experienced so much easier. I was no longer fighting with wondering how to shake things up for dinner because I usually only ate that one meal, and then I would usually only eat what I craved. I would eat until I felt satisfied, and I felt so mentally free! I felt like my inner food demon had gone quiet for once in my life, and I could finally enjoy food without that constant feeling of "missing out" on good foods. Fasting has given me control, and it's helped me get to my lowest weight ever. I feel strong and mentally at peace.

I have done many 23:1 fasts, 47:1 fasts, and even lots of 5:2 fasts (five days fasting, two days eating), but I always try to stay keto as much as I can. I never want my diet to get in the way of my life, but I don't find it hard to find a way to eat keto all the time! My favorite thing to make are keto charcuterie boards!

Something I recommend for anyone wanting to try fasting is to hire a coach. I have a hard time taking care of myself, and I find having an accountability partner/coach to help you makes it so much easier to meet your goals!

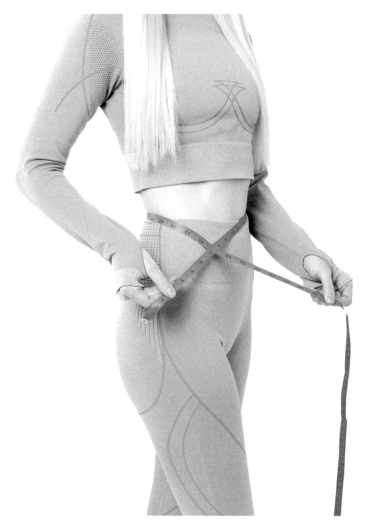

3

THE RECIPES

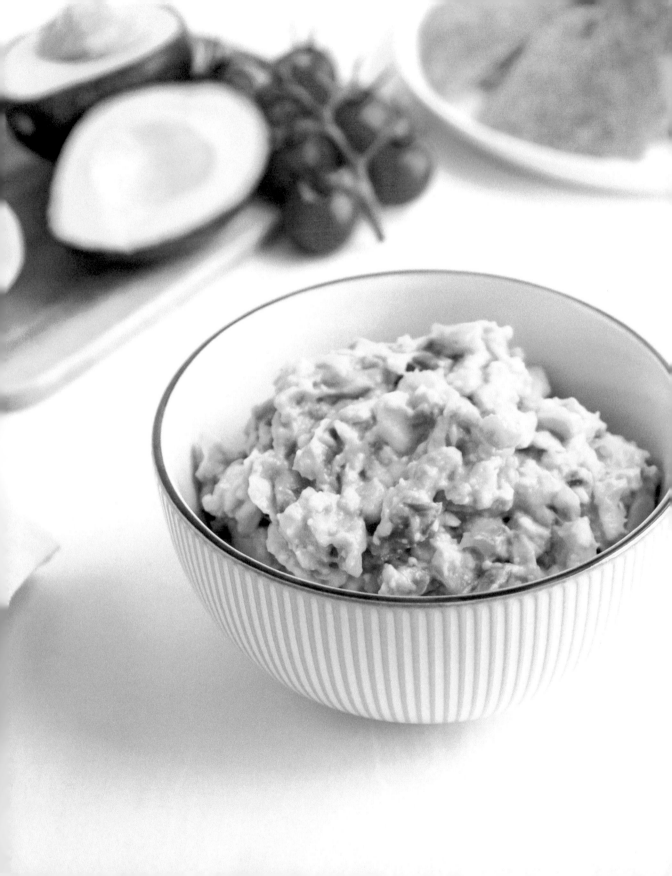

SIDES, SNACKS & SAUCES

BONE BROTH

MAKES about 3 quarts
(8 servings)
PREP TIME: 10 minutes
COOK TIME: 30 minutes, plus 12
to 24 hours in the slow cooker

Bone broth is a fasting essential. It's one of the approved fasting liquids, meaning you can have small sips of bone broth as a crutch on an extended fast (usually seven or more days) if you feel like you would need to break your fast without it and as long as you're not fasting for autophagy. Aside from that, bone broth is also an excellent drink to have in your refeed after a fast.

Bone broth is made by cooking bones and vegetables for several hours. Cooking bone broth for a long time is essential because it takes several hours for all the important minerals and nutrients to be released from the bones. The best bones for making broth include joints, knuckles, marrow bones, oxtail, shank, and short ribs.

2 to 3 pounds animal bones (beef, chicken, pork, or lamb)

2 tablespoons raw, unfiltered apple cider vinegar

2 carrots, cut into large chunks

2 stalks celery, cut into large chunks

1 onion, quartered

1 tablespoon salt

1 teaspoon whole black peppercorns

1. Preheat the oven to 350°F.

2. Place the bones on a roasting tray and roast for 30 minutes, turning halfway through.

3. Transfer the roasted bones to a 5-quart or larger slow cooker and cover with cold water by one inch. Add the vinegar, vegetables, salt, and peppercorns and turn the slow cooker to high.

4. Cover with a lid and cook on high for 1 hour.

5. Lower the heat setting to low and simmer for 12 to 24 hours. The longer you cook your bone broth, the better.

6. Use a large spoon to scoop foam off the surface of the broth once an hour for the first few hours.

7. Once the broth is finished, use a slotted spoon to scoop out the bones and vegetables. Then use a fine-mesh sieve to strain the peppercorns and any remaining bone or vegetable pieces from the broth.

8. Taste the broth and add more salt as needed.

9. The broth can be served right away, or you can place it in the fridge to cool and use later. It will keep in the fridge for five days; you can also freeze it for longer storage (up to three months). Once chilled, the broth will turn to jelly, and there will be a layer of fat on top. You'll be able to scoop and reheat the amount of broth you need. Once reheated, it will reliquefy.

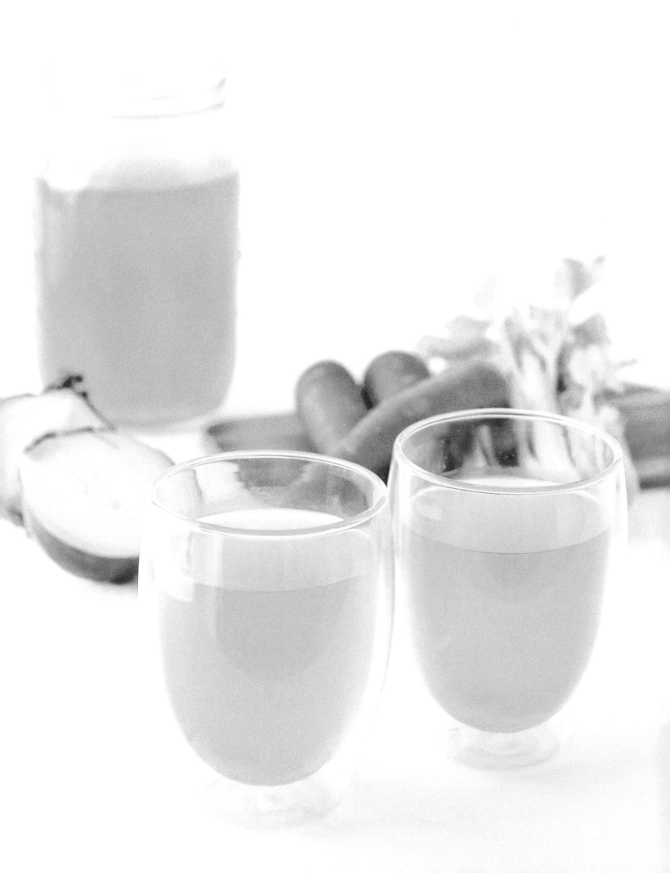

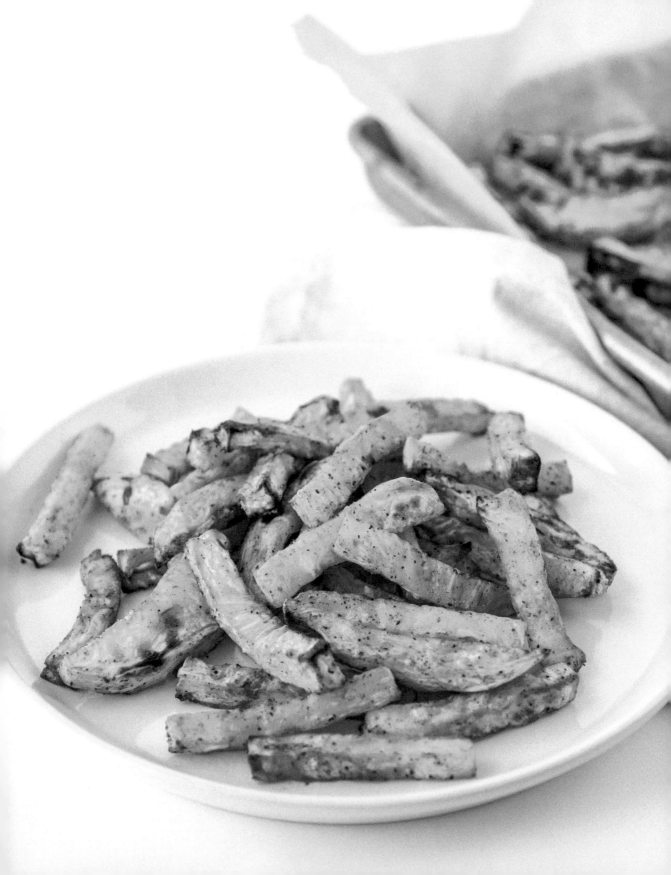

CELERIAC FRIES

SERVES: 2 to 4
PREP TIME: 10 minutes
COOK TIME: 30 minutes

If you've never cooked with celeriac (aka celery root), you've seriously been missing out! You may have walked past it on your supermarket shelf and noticed it because it's kind of an ugly-looking pale lump. But don't be fooled by its lack of beauty! Celeriac is going to be a new delicious staple in your keto kitchen. It basically functions as a replacement potato—most things you would make with potatoes, you can make with celeriac. One of my favorites is fries. You can serve them with any meat of your choice, like beef, pork, chicken, or fish, or just have them on their own sprinkled with salt for a late-night snack.

1 celeriac (aka celery root) (about 2 pounds)

2 tablespoons smoked paprika

1 tablespoon salt

1½ teaspoons ground white pepper

2 tablespoons olive oil

1. Preheat the oven to 400°F on the convection setting. (If you don't have a convection oven, increase the temperature to 430°F.) Line a rimmed baking sheet with parchment paper.

2. Peel the celeriac with a knife, cutting away the outer layer and knobby bits, to reveal the white flesh inside, quarter it, and cut it into ½-inch-wide sticks.

3. In a small bowl, mix the smoked paprika, salt, and white pepper.

4. Put the celeriac sticks in a large bowl, pour in the olive oil, and toss to coat.

5. Spread the celeriac sticks evenly on the prepared baking sheet and sprinkle with the spice mix.

6. Bake for 20 to 30 minutes, until golden brown in color and soft when pierced with a paring knife. Turn the fries halfway through baking.

7. Remove from the oven and serve.

CREAMY CELERIAC BAKE

SERVES: 6
PREP TIME: 10 minutes
COOK TIME: 55 minutes

This creamy celeriac bake is a staple at my house. It works perfectly as a potato dish substitute. (I even prefer it to a potato bake!) Anytime we serve a nice piece of steak or chicken, this bake is our go-to. It can also work as a side dish for brunch with eggs and bacon.

3 tablespoons salted butter, divided

½ onion

3 cloves garlic

2 cups heavy cream

1 tablespoon salt

1 large celeriac (aka celery root) (about 2 pounds)

Shredded cheese like mozzarella or cheddar

1. Preheat the oven to 425°F.

2. Place 2 tablespoons of the butter in a large (approximately 13 by 9-inch) baking dish, then place the dish in the oven until the butter has melted, about 5 minutes.

3. In the meantime, thinly slice the onion and mince the garlic.

4. Melt the remaining tablespoon of butter in a medium skillet over medium heat and cook the onion just until the onion is soft, about five minutes. Do not brown.

5. Take the dish with the melted butter out of the oven and add the minced garlic. Use a pastry brush to coat the inside of the dish with the butter and garlic mixture.

6. Whisk the cream and salt together in a mixing bowl.

7. Use a knife to peel the celeriac, cutting away the outer layer and knobby bits, to reveal the white flesh inside. Then quarter the celeriac and cut into thin slices, or use a food processor with a slicing attachment or mandoline.

8. Layer the celeriac and onion in the prepared dish, then pour in the cream.

9. Place the dish in the middle of the oven and cover loosely with a sheet of aluminum foil. Bake for 30 minutes.

10. Remove from the oven, sprinkle the grated cheese on top, and return to the oven for another 20 minutes, or until the cheese has turned golden brown and the celeriac is soft and cooked through.

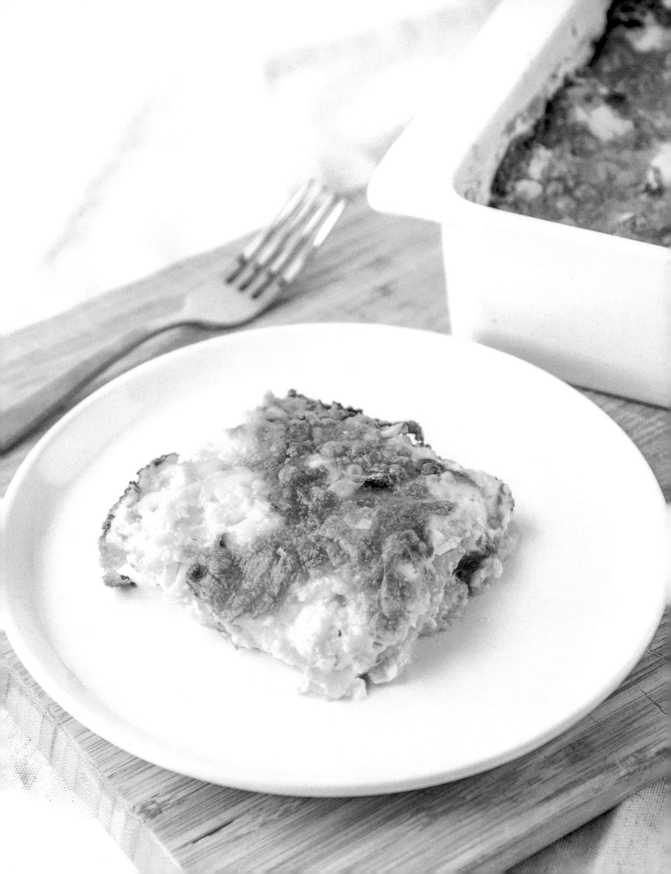

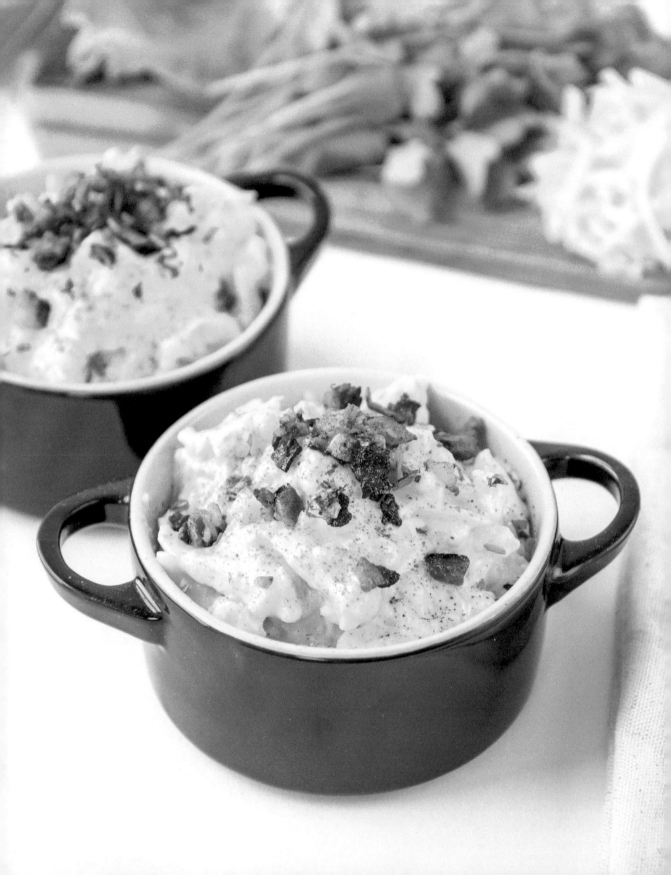

KETO MAC & CHEESE

SERVES: 4
PREP TIME: 8 minutes
COOK TIME: 20 minutes

If you love mac and cheese, you'll love this twist! Instead of using macaroni, this keto version uses small pieces of cauliflower, and let me tell you, it really hits the spot!

Salt

1 large head cauliflower, cut into 1-inch pieces

8 ounces smoked bacon, finely chopped

1¼ cups heavy cream

1 teaspoon paprika

½ to 1 teaspoon turmeric powder (for color)

2 cups shredded cheese like cheddar, mozzarella, and/or Monterey Jack

Ground white pepper

Chopped fresh parsley, for garnish (optional)

1. Bring a large pot of water to a boil and add a large pinch of salt and the cauliflower. Boil until the cauliflower is soft, about 5 minutes; then drain.

2. While the cauliflower is cooking, fry the bacon in a medium skillet over high heat until crispy, about 5 minutes.

3. In a large saucepan, bring the cream, paprika, and turmeric to a simmer over medium heat. Start by adding ½ teaspoon turmeric and check the color. If you want more color, add more turmeric. If you're using yellow cheddar, you may need only a little turmeric.

4. Add the cheese and stir until melted. Then season with salt and white pepper to taste.

5. Add the cauliflower to the cheese sauce and stir until coated.

6. Serve topped with the bacon and parsley, if desired.

CAPRESE SALAD

SERVES: 4
PREP TIME: 10 minutes

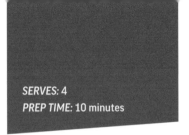

Is there anything fresher and yummier than a caprese salad? Perfect on its own or as a side dish, you can never go wrong with this Italian classic. To keep it keto, make sure you skip the balsamic vinegar.

1 large beefsteak tomato

1 (8-ounce) fresh mozzarella ball

Salt and cracked black pepper

Extra-virgin olive oil

Fresh basil leaves, for garnish

1. Cut the tomato and mozzarella into ½-inch slices and arrange on a plate, alternating the slices of tomato and cheese.

2. Season with salt and cracked black pepper and finish with a drizzle of olive oil.

3. Garnish with fresh basil leaves.

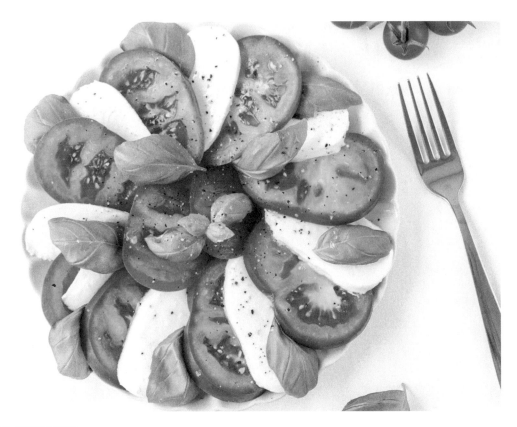

GOUDA CHIPS

SERVES: 4
PREP TIME: 5 minutes
COOK TIME: 15 minutes

If you're looking for a cheesy chip fix, look no further. These Gouda cheese chips are the perfect accompaniment to guac (see page 186 for my recipe). In fact, I don't even miss tortilla chips when I have these around.

8 to 10 deli-style Gouda cheese slices

1 teaspoon paprika

1 teaspoon salt

1. Preheat the oven to 400°F. Line a baking sheet with parchment paper.

2. Cut the cheese slices into quarters on a diagonal and place them on the prepared pan.

3. Season with the paprika and salt, then bake until the cheese has turned golden brown, about 15 minutes.

4. Let cool completely on the baking sheet before removing. Serve immediately.

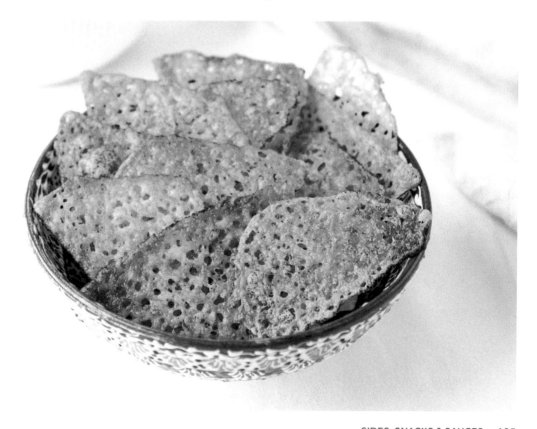

GUACAMOLE

SERVES: 8
PREP TIME: 15 minutes

Everyone has their own twist on guacamole, and this is my favorite. Creamy, fresh, and delicious—this guac will be a hit at your next party. Serve it with chips (page 185), tacos (page 214), or simply as a side dish. Of course, if you're serving four people or fewer, you can always halve this recipe.

4 avocados

4 small tomatoes

4 cloves garlic

Juice of 2 limes

½ teaspoon salt

1. Halve the avocados, remove the pits, and scoop the flesh onto a cutting board.

2. Finely dice the tomatoes and coarsely dice the avocados. Place in a large bowl.

3. Mince or press the garlic cloves and add to the bowl.

4. Add the lime juice and salt, then use a pestle or fork to mash the avocado while mixing to create a creamy texture.

5. Serve immediately.

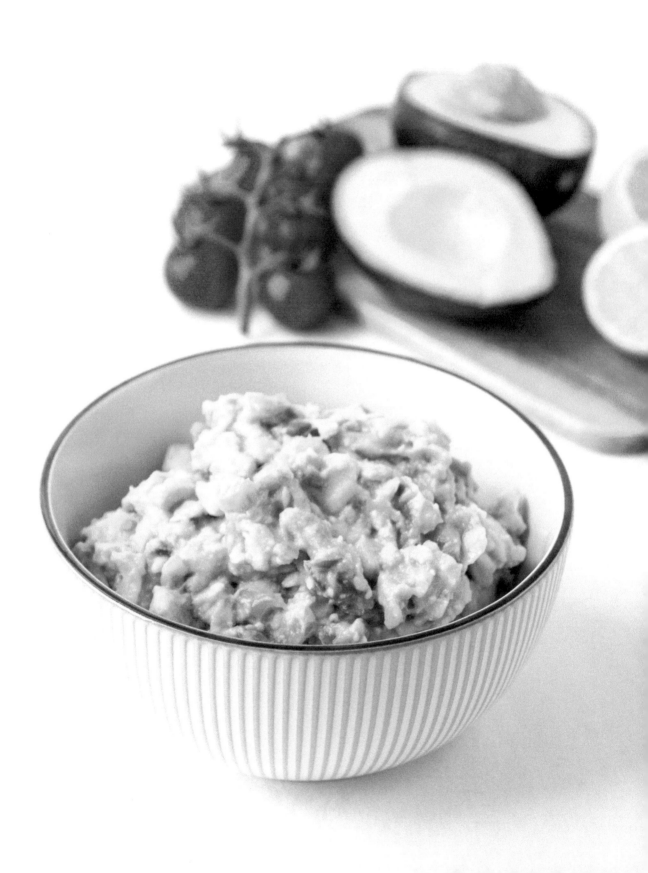

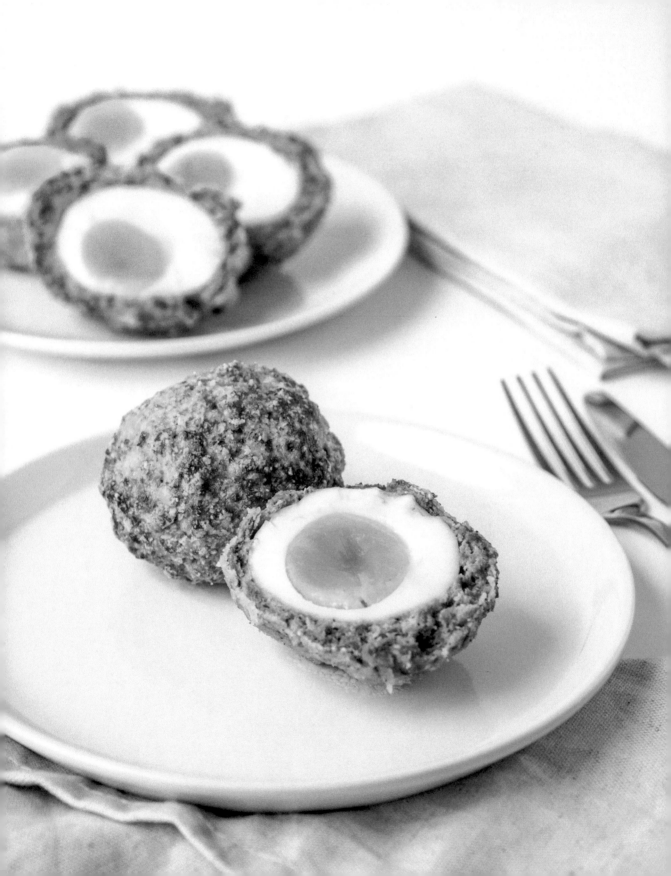

SCOTCH EGGS

SERVES: 4
PREP TIME: 15 minutes
COOK TIME: 20 minutes

This is a British classic that's a perfect on-the-go snack! If you've never tried Scotch eggs, you've really been missing out. They're the perfect mini-meal for the road—creamy eggs covered with savory ground meat. They're a favorite with both adults and kids.

5 large eggs, divided

1 pound ground pork

1 teaspoon salt

1 teaspoon ground black pepper

1 teaspoon dried parsley

1 teaspoon dried sage

1 teaspoon dried thyme

1 cup almond meal

1. Preheat the oven to 450°F. Line a rimmed baking sheet with aluminum foil and place a wire rack over it.

2. Bring a pot of water to a boil and add 4 of the eggs. Boil the eggs for 7 minutes, then place in a bowl of cold water to stop the cooking.

3. Mix the ground pork with the salt, pepper, and herbs in a medium mixing bowl.

4. Peel the eggs and divide the meat mixture into four equal portions, then form each portion into a ball. Flatten a ball of meat into a thin patty, place an egg in the middle, and then cover the egg with the meat; press the edges together to seal. Make sure the whole egg is evenly covered or you'll risk the eggs splitting in the oven.

5. Whisk the remaining egg in a small bowl and place the almond meal in a separate bowl.

6. Dip the meat-covered eggs into the egg, then into the almond meal and coat completely.

7. Place on the wire rack and bake for 15 to 20 minutes, until the meat coating is golden brown. Remove from the oven and allow to rest for 5 to 10 minutes. Serve warm or allow to cool to room temperature before serving. Store leftovers in the fridge for up to 4 days.

CREAMY MUSHROOM GRAVY

SERVES: 6
PREP TIME: 5 minutes
COOK TIME: 12 minutes

Looking for a tasty and versatile sauce for almost any dish? This rich, garlicky mushroom gravy is the solution. Flavor tip: If you're cooking this sauce to serve with steak, chicken, pork, or other pan-fried protein, remove the meat from the pan and cook the sauce in the same pan to utilize the meat juices. If you're making this sauce on its own, proceed with the recipe as written.

1 tablespoon salted butter

1 (8-ounce) package sliced mushrooms

2 cloves garlic, minced

2 cups heavy cream

Salt and pepper

Leaves from 2 sprigs fresh parsley, finely chopped

1. Heat a medium skillet over high heat. Melt the butter in the hot pan and then add the mushrooms and garlic and cook until the mushrooms have softened and reduced in size, about 5 minutes.

2. Pour in the cream, season generously with salt and pepper, and bring to a simmer.

3. Simmer until the sauce has thickened, about 5 minutes and then remove from the heat. Stir in the parsley before serving. This sauce can be stored in the fridge in an airtight container for up to 4 days.

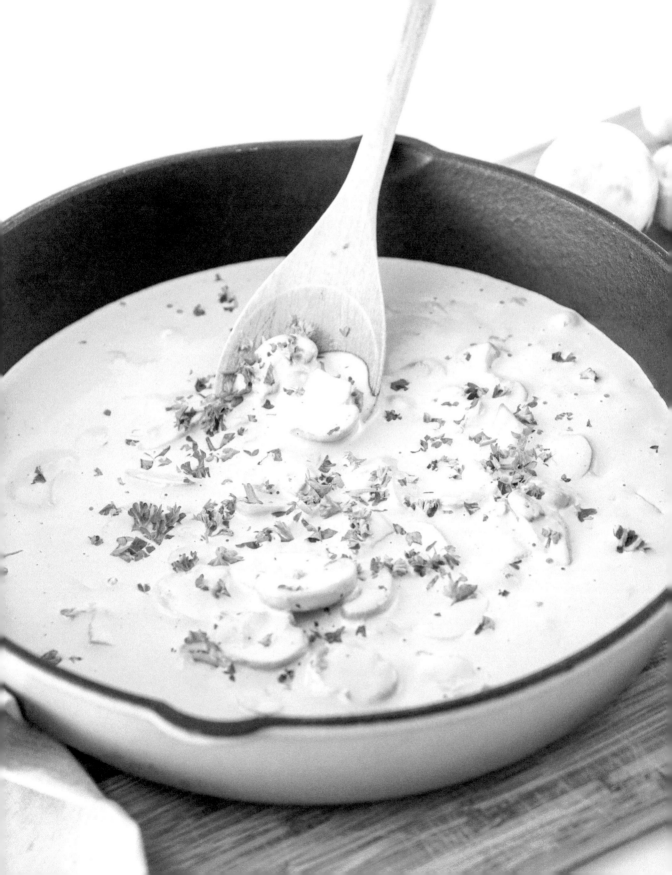

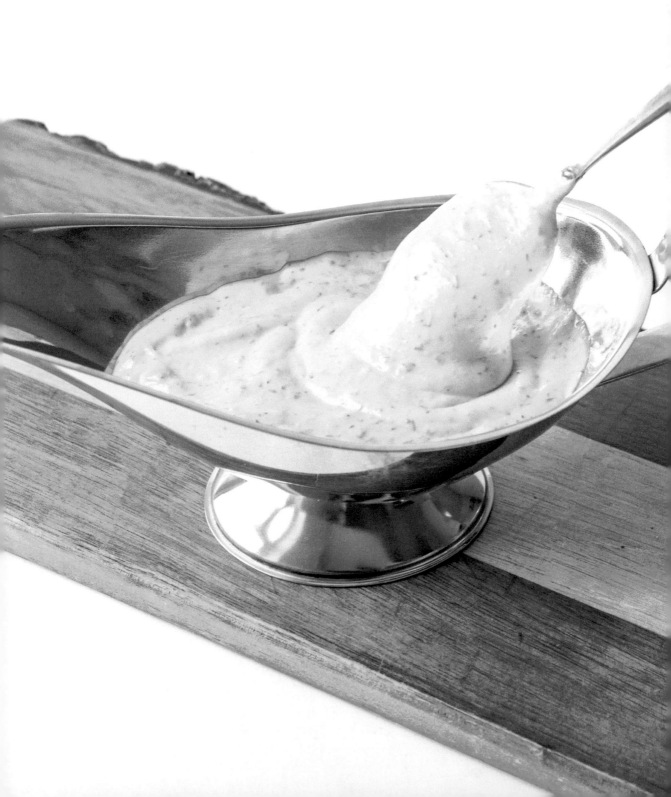

BÉARNAISE SAUCE

SERVES: 6
PREP TIME: 5 minutes
COOK TIME: 20 minutes

Béarnaise sauce is one of the tastiest sauces to use as an accompaniment for steak, and it goes equally well with chicken or pork. This traditional French sauce can be a bit tricky to make because it's an emulsion, which means you have to be vigilant to prepare sure it doesn't split. But fear not! I've found a foolproof way to make it. The key is to use an immersion blender and a tall container instead of making it the classic way by whisking it over a double boiler. Impress your friends with this restaurant-quality sauce in just under 30 minutes.

4 sprigs fresh tarragon

½ cup dry white wine

¼ cup white wine vinegar

1 small shallot, chopped

10 whole black peppercorns

12 tablespoons (1½ sticks) salted butter

2 large egg yolks

SPECIAL EQUIPMENT:

Immersion blender and a tall container

1. Separate the tarragon leaves from the stems. Set the stems aside and finely chop the leaves.

2. In a small saucepan over high heat, stir together the tarragon stems, wine, vinegar, shallot, and peppercorns. Bring to a boil, then lower the heat to medium and simmer until the liquid has reduced to about 3 tablespoons, about 10 minutes.

3. Pour the wine reduction through a fine mesh sieve into a tall container that barely fits the head of an immersion blender. Use a spoon to press the solids to extract as much of the liquid as possible. Set aside.

4. Using the same saucepan, melt the butter over high heat until the foaming subsides, about 1 minute. Remove the pan from the heat.

5. Add the egg yolks and the tarragon leaves to the container with the wine reduction.

6. Use the immersion blender to blend the egg and wine mixture while slowly pouring in the melted butter. Move the blender head up and down in the mixture while blending. The sauce should be thick and creamy.

7. Serve immediately, or let cool and allow to sit for up to 2 hours before serving. Note: This sauce cannot be stored in the fridge and reheated.

TZATZIKI

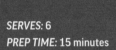

SERVES: 6
PREP TIME: 15 minutes

Tzatziki is a huge summer favorite at my house! It works with practically any protein—pork, steak, chicken, lamb, or fish—and is a great way to add some freshness to your plate.

1 English cucumber (aka greenhouse or European cucumber)

1 teaspoon salt

2 cups full-fat Greek yogurt

3 cloves garlic, minced

Juice of 1 lemon

1 tablespoon extra-virgin olive oil

1. Using the large holes on a box grater, shred the cucumber. Place in a fine-mesh sieve and mix with the salt. Leave to drain for 5 minutes.

2. In a large bowl, combine the yogurt, garlic, and lemon juice.

3. Using your hands or a rubber spatula, gently press any remaining juice from the cucumber, then add the cucumber to the yogurt mixture and stir to combine.

4. Drizzle the olive oil over the tzatziki and serve immediately, or store in an airtight container in the fridge for up to 4 days.

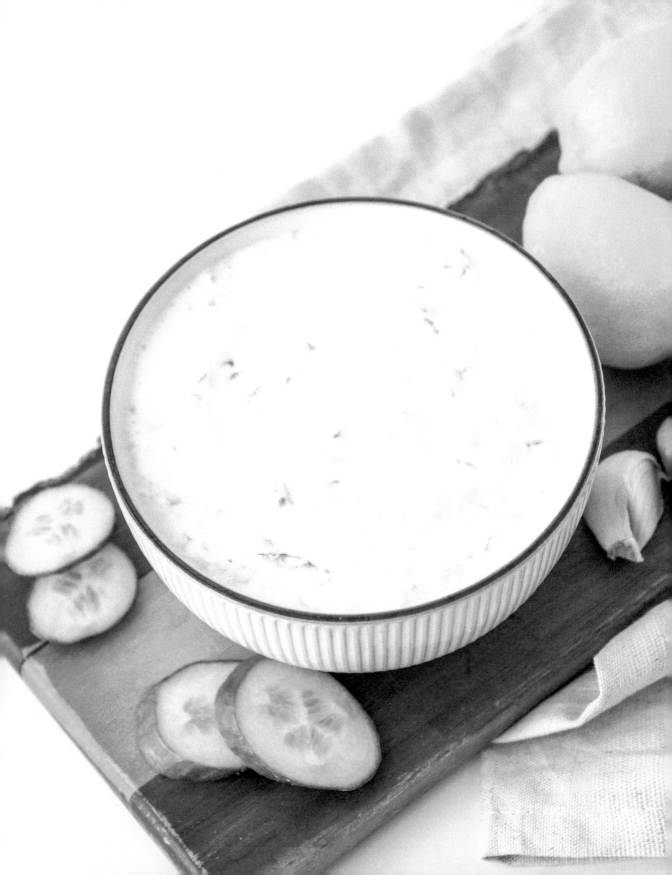

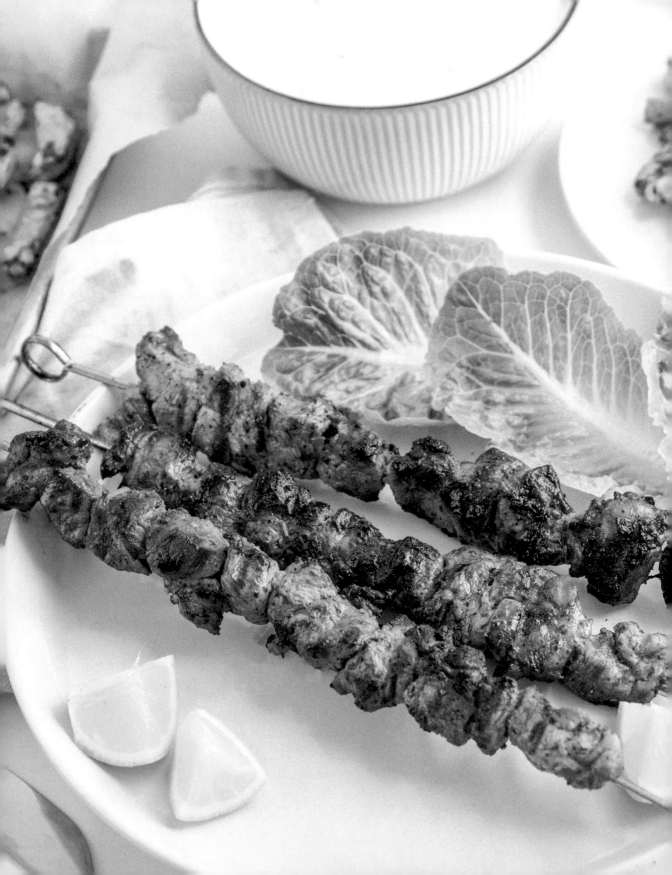

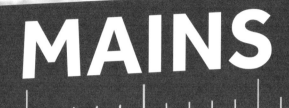

MAINS

CRACK SLAW

SERVES: 4
PREP TIME: 10 minutes
COOK TIME: 25 minutes

This is one of my favorite quick and easy midweek keto meals. Crack slaw got its name due to how addictively delicious it is, and I can confirm that the rumors are true! I usually make crack slaw with ground pork, but the recipe is super versatile. You can use any (preferably high-fat) ground protein you choose, so feel free to swap in beef, chicken, or turkey.

2 tablespoons toasted sesame oil

1 pound ground pork, beef, chicken, or turkey

4 cloves garlic, minced

1 medium head cabbage, finely sliced

2 tablespoons soy sauce

2 teaspoons apple cider vinegar

½ teaspoon erythritol or stevia (optional)

1 teaspoon salt

1 teaspoon ground black pepper

4 to 5 green onions, chopped, plus more for garnish

1 tablespoon toasted sesame seeds, for garnish

1. Heat the sesame oil in a large skillet over high heat. Add the ground meat and sauté until cooked through, about 10 minutes.

2. Mix in the garlic and fry for 2 to 3 minutes, until it's soft and translucent.

3. Add the cabbage to the skillet and mix in.

4. Add the soy sauce, vinegar, sweetener (if using), salt, and pepper. Fry for another 5 minutes, or until the cabbage is cooked to your liking.

5. Mix in the green onions and fry for 2 more minutes, until they are slightly wilted.

6. Plate, then sprinkle with the toasted sesame seeds.

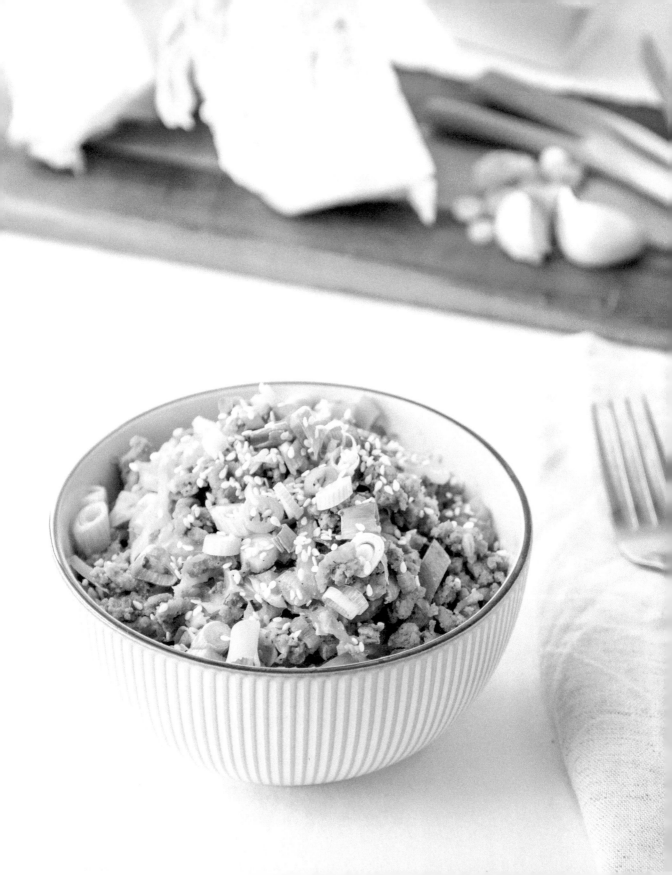

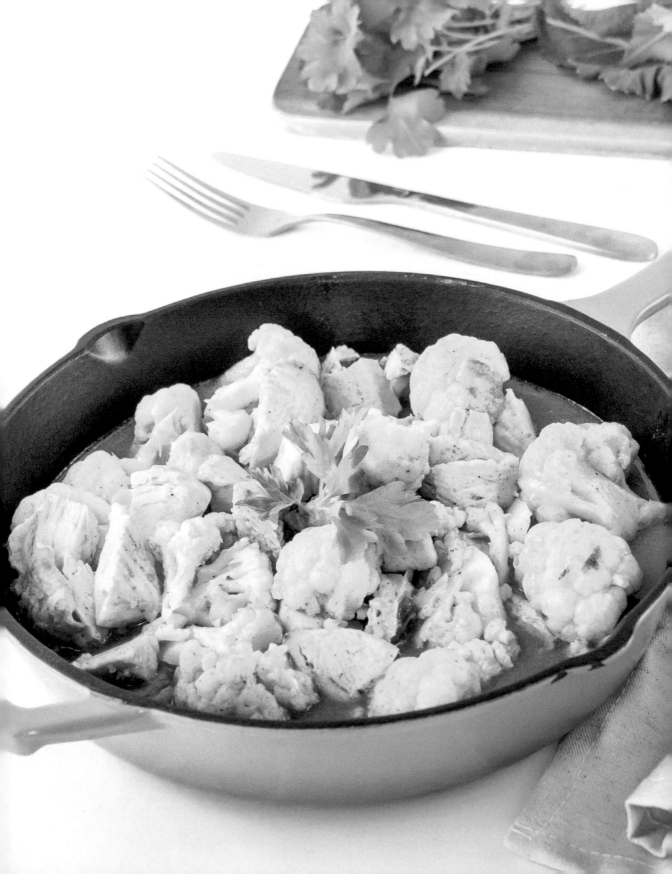

CHICKEN CAULIFLOWER CURRY

SERVES: 4 to 6
PREP TIME: 10 minutes
COOK TIME: 25 minutes

If you're looking for a one-pot-wonder dish, look no further! This creamy curry is perfect for cozy fall and winter nights because of the warmth coming from the spice mix of cumin, turmeric, and coriander. This curry also has the benefit of being super quick to make!

1 (13.5-ounce) can full-fat coconut milk

1 teaspoon ground cumin

1 teaspoon turmeric powder

1 teaspoon ground coriander

1 teaspoon salt

1 large cauliflower head, cut into large florets

1 pound boneless, skinless chicken breasts, cut into 2-inch pieces

Fresh flat-leaf parsley, for garnish (optional)

1. Bring the coconut milk, spices, and salt to a simmer in a large skillet over medium heat.

2. Add the cauliflower, cover with a lid, and simmer for 10 minutes, stirring occasionally.

3. Add the chicken and simmer for another 10 minutes, or until the chicken is cooked through and the cauliflower is soft. Garnish with parsley before serving, if desired.

FISH SOUP

SERVES: 4
PREP TIME: 5 minutes
COOK TIME: 15 minutes

This is another simple dish that is so comforting. The soup brings together a tasty mix of different fish in a smooth tomato-based broth. It's the perfect warming meal to pull together in less than half an hour.

1 tablespoon salted butter

½ medium onion, finely chopped

1 (14-ounce) can crushed tomatoes

1 cup fish stock

1 cup heavy whipping cream

1 pound mixed fish fillets (such as salmon, cod, and haddock), cut into 2-inch pieces

Salt

Chopped fresh parsley, for garnish

1. Put the butter in a large pot and set over high heat.

2. When the butter has melted, add the onion and cook until translucent.

3. Add the tomatoes, stock, and cream and bring to a simmer.

4. Add the fish and simmer for 5 minutes, or until the fish is cooked through (it should flake easily when done).

5. Salt to taste. Garnish with chopped parsley before serving.

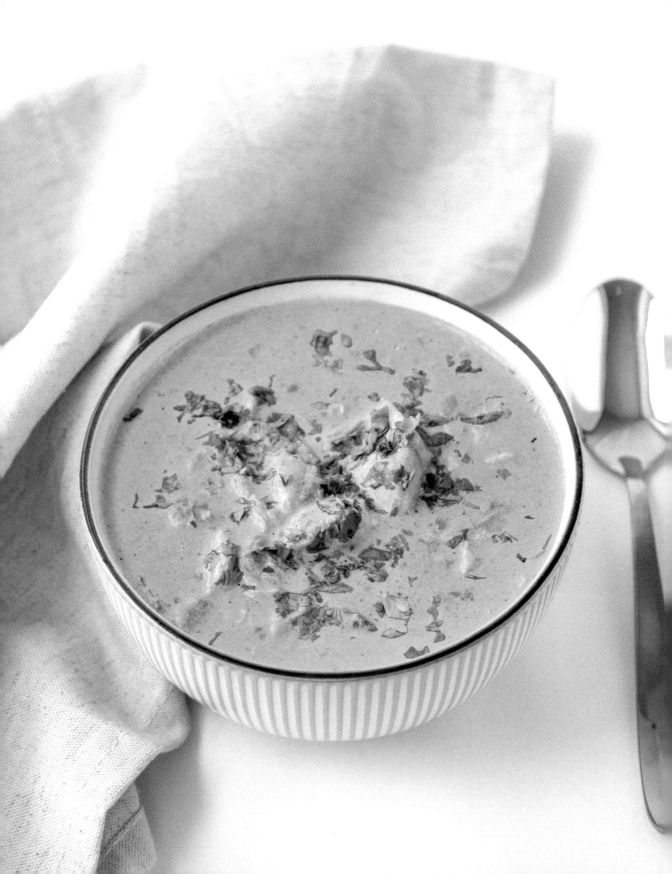

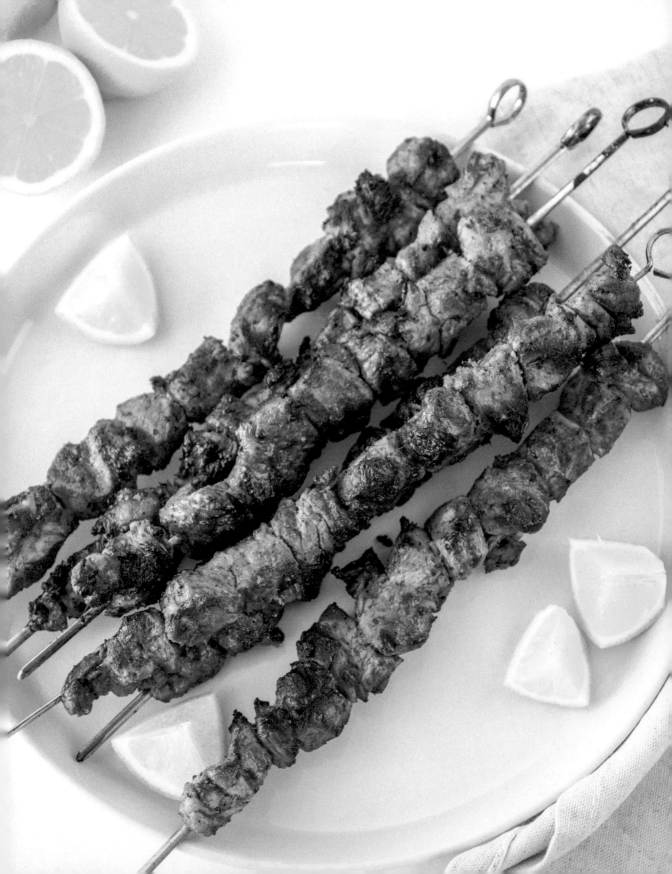

PORK SOUVLAKI

SERVES: 4
PREP TIME: 15 minutes
COOK TIME: 10 minutes

This Greek-inspired pork souvlaki is the perfect summer dish. I love making it on the grill, but if you don't have one, you can easily make it in the oven using the broiler. For a truly satisfying and impressive meal, try serving these skewers with Celeriac Fries (page 179) and Tzatziki (page 194).

FOR THE MARINADE:

1 tablespoon extra-virgin olive oil

1 tablespoon ground dried oregano

1½ teaspoons paprika

1½ teaspoons ground cumin

1 teaspoon salt

Juice of 1 lemon

1 pound boneless pork shoulder, cut into 2-inch cubes

FOR SERVING:

2 heads little gem or baby romaine lettuce, separated into leaves

Lemon wedges

SPECIAL EQUIPMENT:

Four 12-inch metal skewers

1. Mix the oil, spices, salt, and lemon juice in a bowl. Add the meat and toss to coat until completely covered by the marinade.

2. If cooking in the oven, line a sheet pan with parchment paper, place an oven rack in the middle of the oven, and preheat the broiler to high. If cooking on an outdoor grill, preheat the grill to high.

3. Thread the marinated pork pieces onto the skewers.

4. If using the oven, place the skewers on the prepared sheet pan and bake for 4 to 5 minutes; then flip over and bake for 4 to 5 minutes more. Alternatively, place the skewers on the grill and cook for about 10 minutes, turning occasionally. The meat is done when golden brown on the outside and no longer pink on the inside.

5. Serve with lettuce leaves as wraps and lemon wedges.

CABBAGE LASAGNA

SERVES: 4
PREP TIME: 15 minutes
COOK TIME: 60 minutes

When you're craving Italian but pasta is out of the question, this cabbage lasagna really hits the spot. In fact, this lasagna is so good that I prefer it to traditional lasagna.

1 tablespoon salted butter

1 tablespoon extra-virgin olive oil

½ medium onion, finely chopped

1 pound ground pork

1 (14-ounce) can crushed tomatoes

1 cup beef broth, homemade (page 176) or store bought

1 tablespoon Italian seasoning

2 teaspoons salt

1 teaspoon ground black pepper

1 large head cabbage

1 cup shredded mozzarella or cheddar cheese

FOR THE WHITE SAUCE:

1 tablespoon salted butter

1 teaspoon xanthan gum

2 cups heavy cream

1 teaspoon salt

1 teaspoon ground white pepper

Chopped fresh basil leaves, for garnish

1. Heat the butter and oil in a large skillet over high heat.

2. Add the onion and fry for 1 minute, until softened.

3. Add the ground pork and brown, crumbling the meat as it cooks.

4. Add the tomatoes, broth, Italian seasoning, salt, and pepper and bring to a boil. Reduce the heat and simmer until the liquid has reduced by half, about 15 minutes, then remove the pan from the heat.

5. While the sauce is simmering, prepare the cabbage: Bring a large pot of water to a boil. Cut the bottom off the cabbage head and quarter.

6. Once the water is boiling, add a large pinch of salt and gently drop in the cabbage quarters. Boil for 10 minutes, then drain and set aside until cool enough to handle.

7. To prepare the white sauce, heat the butter in a medium pot over high heat.

8. Once the butter has melted and starts to simmer, take off the heat and whisk in the xanthan gum. Gradually pour in the cream while whisking constantly and return to the heat.

9. Season with the salt and pepper, then bring to a boil while whisking until the sauce has thickened, about 2 minutes.

10. To assemble and bake, preheat the oven to 400°F. Pull apart the cooled cabbage leaves. Layer the meat sauce, cabbage leaves, and white sauce in a 13 by 9-inch baking dish. Top with the shredded cheese. Place the dish in the middle of the oven and bake for 30 minutes, or until the cheese has turned golden brown. Allow to sit for about 15 minutes before serving. Garnish with chopped basil.

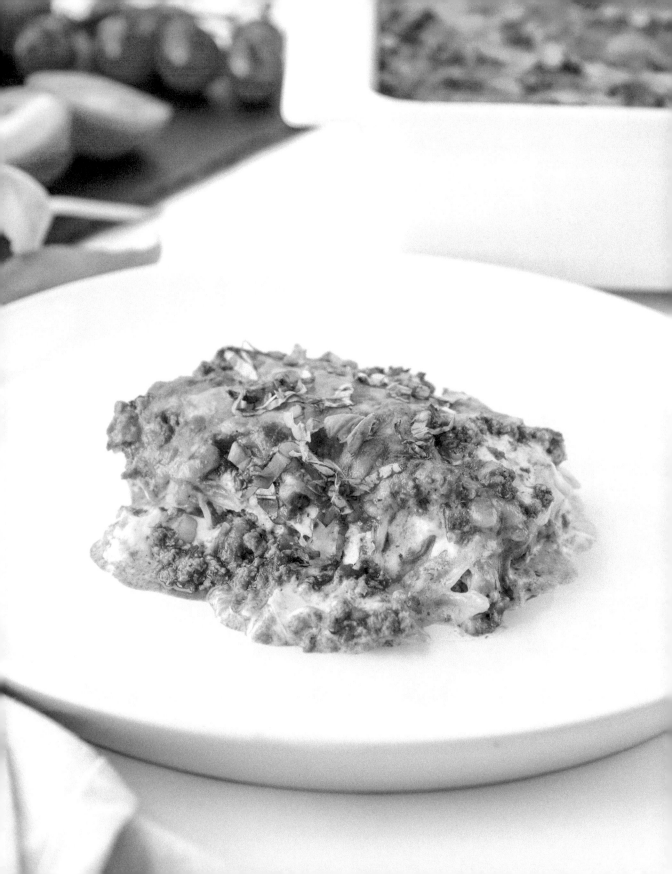

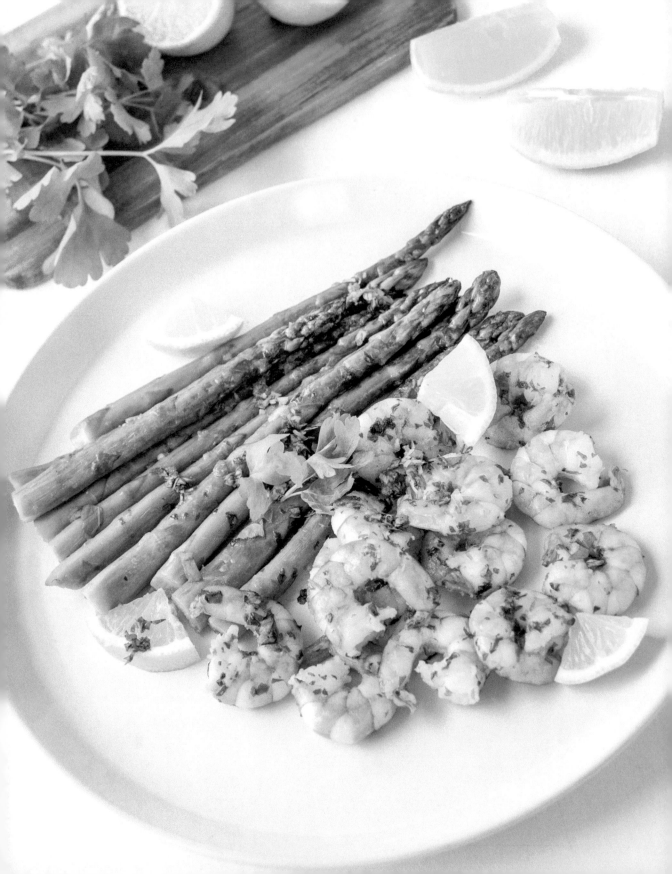

GARLIC BUTTER SHRIMP & ASPARAGUS

SERVES: 4
PREP TIME: 10 minutes
COOK TIME: 10 minutes

This dish is so easy to throw together. It's also incredibly tasty and gives me those Mediterranean summer vibes!

1 tablespoon extra-virgin olive oil

1 tablespoon salted butter

3 cloves garlic, minced

1 pound medium-thick asparagus, tough ends snapped off

1 pound large shrimp, peeled and deveined

Juice of ½ lemon

¼ cup chopped fresh parsley, plus more for garnish if desired

Pinch of salt

Lemon wedges, for serving

1. Heat the olive oil and butter in a large skillet over high heat until simmering.

2. Add the garlic and asparagus and cook for 5 minutes, turning occasionally.

3. Add the shrimp, lemon juice, parsley, and salt and cook, turning occasionally, for 2 minutes, or until the shrimp are opaque and have become pink or orange. Garnish with parsley, if desired, and serve with lemon wedges.

BROCCOLI & CAULIFLOWER SOUP with BACON SPRINKLES

SERVES: 8
PREP TIME: 10 minutes
COOK TIME: 25 minutes

This soup is one of my all-time favorite recipes. It is creamy and hearty and hits the spot perfectly when you're looking for a warm and comforting meal.

2 tablespoons salted butter

½ medium onion, diced

4 cloves garlic, minced

1 large head broccoli, florets and stem, chopped

½ medium head cauliflower, chopped

2 medium zucchinis, chopped

2 cups vegetable broth

2 teaspoons salt

2 teaspoons ground black pepper

2 cups heavy cream

8 ounces thick-cut smoked bacon, finely diced

1. Melt the butter in a large pot over high heat, then sauté the onion and garlic until soft.

2. Add the broccoli, cauliflower, and zucchini to the pot along with the broth, salt, and pepper. Cover with a lid, turn the heat to medium, and simmer for 15 minutes, or until soft.

3. While the vegetables are cooking, fry the bacon over high heat in a separate skillet until golden and slightly crispy, about 5 minutes. Use a slotted spoon to transfer the bacon to a bowl and set aside.

4. When the vegetables are soft, pour in the cream and simmer for 5 minutes.

5. Use an immersion blender to partially blend the soup in the pot to give it a creamier texture. If you do not have an immersion blender, you can transfer the soup to a regular blender and pulse for a few seconds until the soup has a creamier texture. The soup should not be completely smooth.

6. Serve the soup with the bacon sprinkled on top.

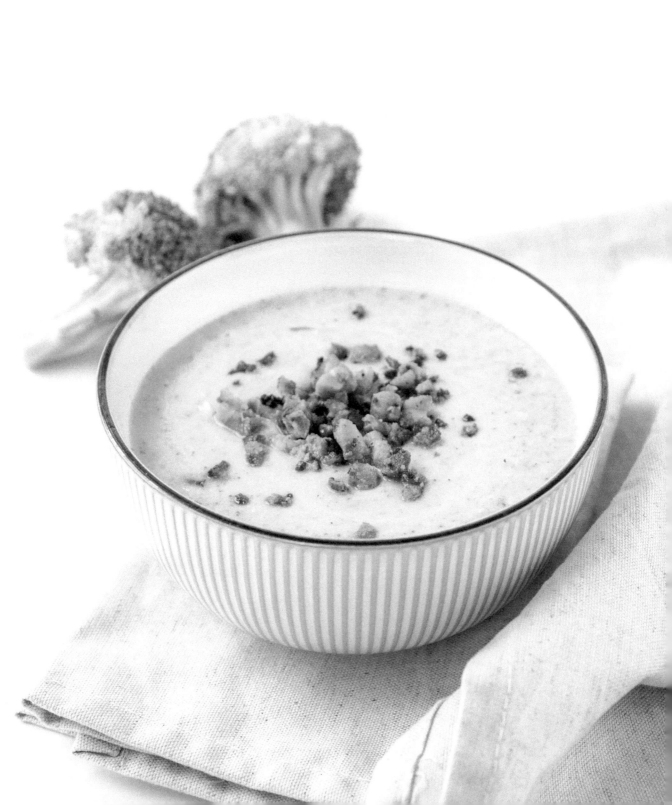

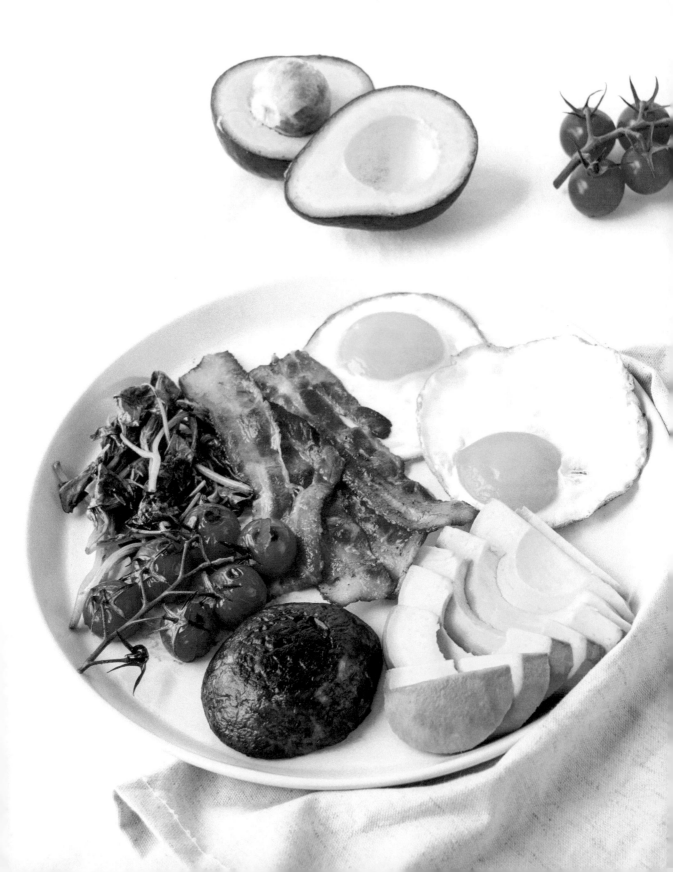

KETO ENGLISH BREAKFAST

SERVES: 4
PREP TIME: 5 minutes
COOK TIME: 15 minutes

A real English classic! The traditional English breakfast usually comes with hash browns, baked beans, and toast, but in this keto version, I have swapped all of that for delicious keto-friendly avocado and sautéed spinach.

8 to 12 slices smoked bacon

2 tablespoons salted butter, divided

24 cherry tomatoes

4 medium portobello mushrooms

8 cups fresh baby spinach

4 avocados

8 large eggs

Salt and pepper

1. Fry the bacon in a large skillet over high heat until done to your liking.

2. In a separate skillet, melt 1 tablespoon of the butter over medium heat, then fry the tomatoes and mushrooms until the tomatoes are beginning to shrivel and the mushrooms are browned.

3. In a separate large skillet, fry the spinach over medium heat until wilted, stirring occasionally.

4. Slice the avocados.

5. Melt the remaining tablespoon of butter in a large skillet over medium heat. Working in two batches, fry the eggs to your liking, season with a pinch of salt and pepper, and serve, dividing everything evenly among 4 plates.

TACO LETTUCE WRAPS

SERVES: 4
PREP TIME: 10 minutes
COOK TIME: 10 minutes

I love tacos, and swapping the tortilla for a lettuce wrap is the perfect way to get your taco fix while following a keto way of eating. I like lots of toppings on my tacos, but you can pick your favorites among the topping ideas listed below; for the guacamole, see my recipe on page 186.

1 tablespoon salted butter

1 pound ground pork or beef

1 teaspoon ground cumin

1 teaspoon paprika

1 teaspoon ground black pepper

1 teaspoon salt

8 to 12 gem lettuce or baby romaine leaves

SUGGESTED TOPPINGS:

Diced cucumbers

Diced tomatoes or quartered cherry tomatoes

Sour cream

Salsa

Sliced avocado or guacamole

Shredded cheese

1. Melt the butter in a large skillet over high heat, then add the ground meat.

2. Fry for a couple of minutes, stirring to break up the meat. Add the spices and salt and continue to fry until cooked through (the meat will no longer be pink at the center when fully cooked).

3. Cut the bottoms off the lettuce leaves and separate the leaves.

4. Serve the taco meat in the lettuce wraps with your favorite toppings.

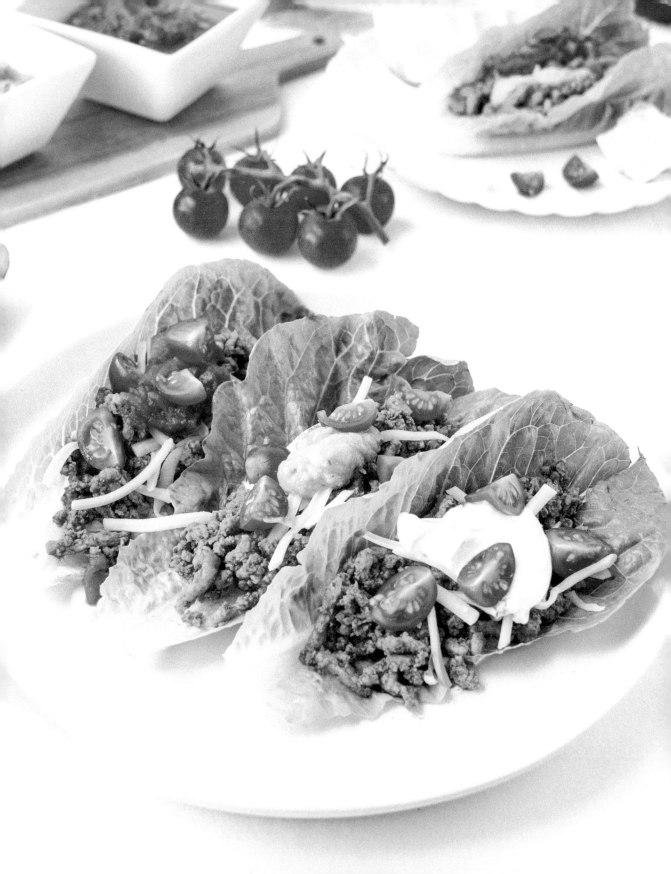

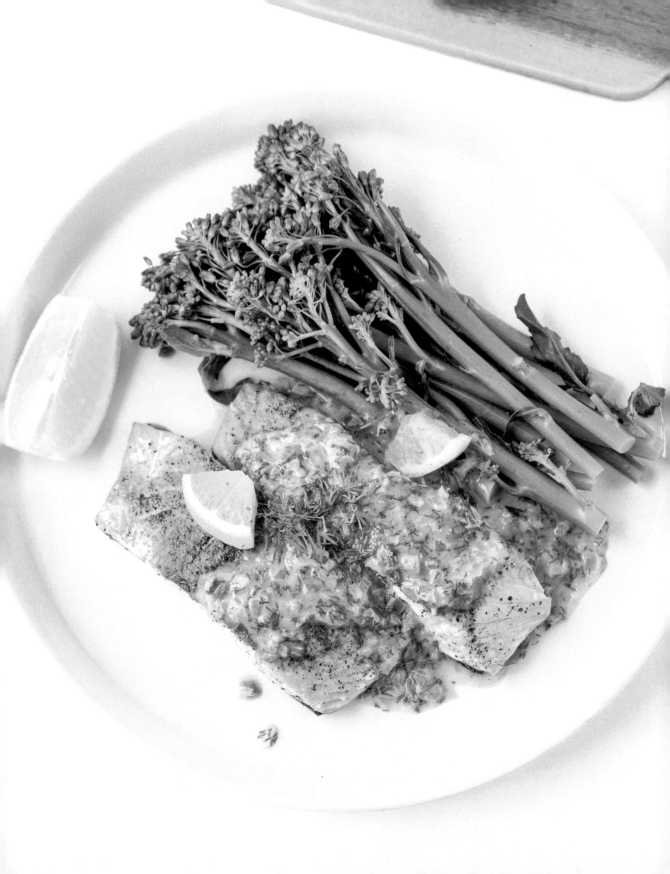

SALMON with BROCCOLINI & LEMON HERB SAUCE

SERVES: 4
PREP TIME: 10 minutes
COOK TIME: 25 minutes

I love salmon however it's prepared, but this is my favorite salmon recipe. It's super fresh and summery, and the lemon and herb sauce is to die for!

4 (4.5-ounce) skin-on salmon fillets, about 1½ inches thick

Salt and pepper

1 tablespoon salted butter

1 pound broccolini

FOR THE SAUCE:

2 tablespoons salted butter, divided

2 shallots, finely diced

4 sprigs fresh dill, finely chopped

Juice of 1 lemon

2 cups chicken broth

Lemon wedges, for serving

1. Generously season the salmon with salt and pepper on both sides.

2. Heat the butter in a large skillet over medium heat until simmering, then add the salmon and cook, skin side down, for 6 minutes; then turn and cook on the other side for 6 minutes more, or until the fish is cooked through, opaque and glistening in the middle.

3. While the fish is cooking, prepare the broccolini: Bring a large pot of salted water to a boil, then carefully drop in the broccolini. Boil for 5 minutes, until soft, then drain.

4. To make the sauce, melt 1 tablespoon of the butter in a medium saucepan over high heat, then add the shallots and fry until soft.

5. Add the lemon juice, dill, and broth and simmer rapidly until the liquid has reduced by half.

6. Remove the pan from the heat, add the remaining tablespoon of butter, and stir until melted.

7. Plate the salmon with the sauce on top and the broccolini on the side.

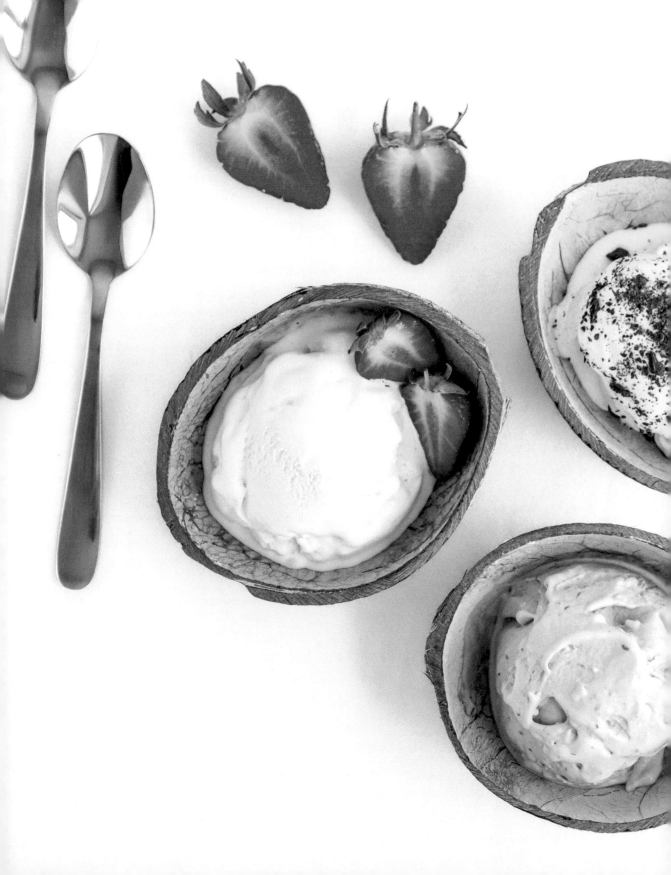

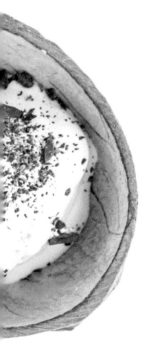

DESSERTS

KETO MUD CAKE

SERVES: 8 to 10
PREP TIME: 10 minutes, plus at least 1 hour to chill
COOK TIME: 20 minutes

This keto mud cake is a favorite at my house! It's a keto twist on kladdkaka, a sticky chocolate cake I grew up with in Sweden. It's super rich and gooey—kind of like a brownie but better. Traditionally it's served with whipped cream and strawberries. It's simple but delicious.

10 tablespoons (1¼ sticks) salted butter, plus 1 tablespoon for the pan

100 grams blanched almond flour

3 large eggs

⅔ cup powdered erythritol

1 teaspoon baking powder

1 teaspoon vanilla extract

¼ cup cacao powder, plus 1½ teaspoons for the pan

Pinch of salt

FOR SERVING (OPTIONAL):

1½ cups heavy cream

1 tablespoon powdered erythritol

Sliced fresh strawberries

SPECIAL EQUIPMENT:

9-inch springform pan

1. Preheat the oven to 350°F. Grease the springform pan with 1 tablespoon of butter, then coat the greased pan with 1½ teaspoons of cacao power.

2. Melt the remaining butter in a small saucepan over medium heat.

3. Use an electric mixer on medium speed to whisk the melted butter, almond flour, eggs, erythritol, baking powder, vanilla extract, cacao powder, and salt until thoroughly combined.

4. Pour the batter into the prepared pan and spread out evenly. Bake for 15 to 19 minutes, until the middle part of the cake still moves but the edges are set. Not overbaking the cake is crucial to ensure that it has the right stickiness. Open the oven door and check the cake by gently shaking the pan.

5. Remove from the oven, allow to cool to room temperature, and then place in the fridge to chill for at least 1 hour.

6. Pour the cream into a bowl and whip with a mixer until stiff peaks form.

7. Remove the sides of the springform pan and use a fine-mesh sieve to sprinkle the erythritol over the cake. Slice and serve with the whipped cream and strawberries, if desired.

8. Store leftovers in an airtight container in the fridge for up to 4 days.

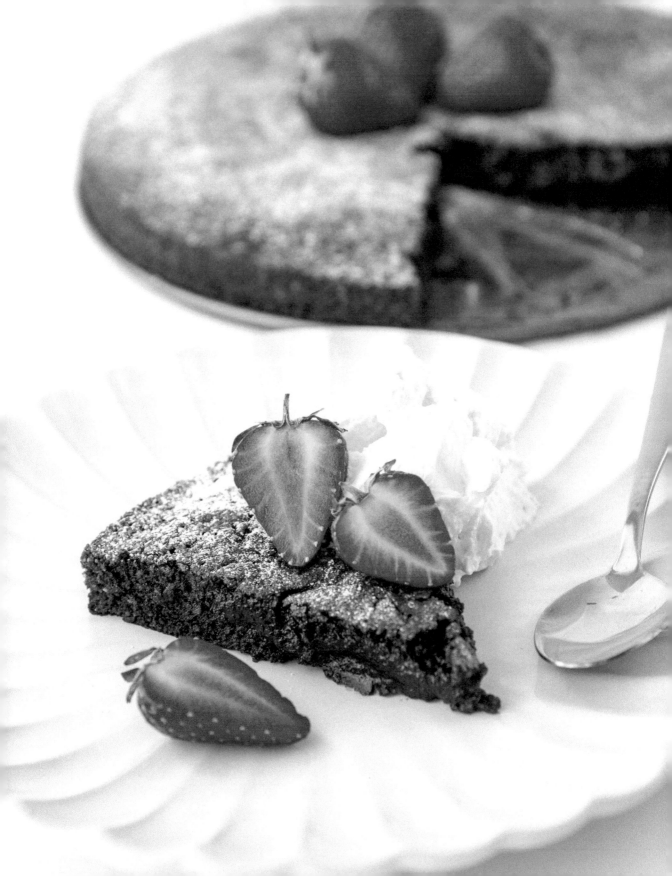

KETO ICE CREAM

SERVES: 6
PREP TIME: 5 minutes + 4 hrs+ to chill the base + 30 mins–6 hrs to churn (depending on method)
COOK TIME: 45 minutes

This ice cream is rich, creamy, and easy to make at home. The secret to getting the perfect keto ice cream is making your own condensed milk first. It's a game changer for getting a smooth and velvety texture. Chilling the ice cream base in the fridge overnight before churning also makes a big difference. And don't worry if you don't have an ice cream maker! I offer two methods in this recipe: one uses an ice cream maker and the other doesn't require one. You can customize your ice cream by adding mix-ins like berries, nuts, or cacao nibs.

3 tablespoons salted butter

⅓ cup powdered erythritol

3 cups heavy cream, divided

2 teaspoons vanilla extract

1 cup unsweetened, unflavored almond milk

¼ cup MCT oil

OPTIONAL MIX-INS:

Blueberries

Raspberries

Strawberries

Cacao nibs

100% dark chocolate pieces

Unsweetened coconut flakes

Chopped hazelnuts

OPTIONAL TOPPING:

Cocoa powder or ground cinnamon

SPECIAL EQUIPMENT (optional):

Ice cream maker

1. Make the condensed milk: Melt the butter in a medium saucepan over medium heat; do not allow it to come to a simmer or to brown. Add the erythritol and 2 cups of the cream to the pan. Bring the mixture to a low boil, then reduce the heat and simmer gently, stirring frequently, for 30 to 45 minutes, until the mixture is thick (like condensed milk) and coats the back of a spoon. Once sufficiently thickened, the volume should have reduced by half.

2. Make the ice cream base: Pour the condensed milk into a bowl and set in an ice bath. Allow to cool to room temperature, then mix in the vanilla extract.

3. Add the almond milk, MCT oil, and remaining cup of heavy cream and whisk until smooth.

4. Cover with plastic wrap and place the ice cream base in the fridge to chill for at least 4 hours or overnight.

5. *If using an ice cream maker,* transfer the base to the ice cream maker and churn following the manufacturer's instructions until the ice cream reaches soft-serve consistency, usually about 30 minutes. If you want to add mix-ins, add them toward the end of the churning process. If adding berries, puree them in a blender before adding to the ice cream. Transfer the ice cream to a freezer-safe container and freeze for 2 to 4 hours, until firm.

   If not using an ice cream maker, transfer the base to a 2-quart freezer-safe container. Line the surface with a parchment paper to keep ice crystals from forming. Freeze for 4 to 6 hours,

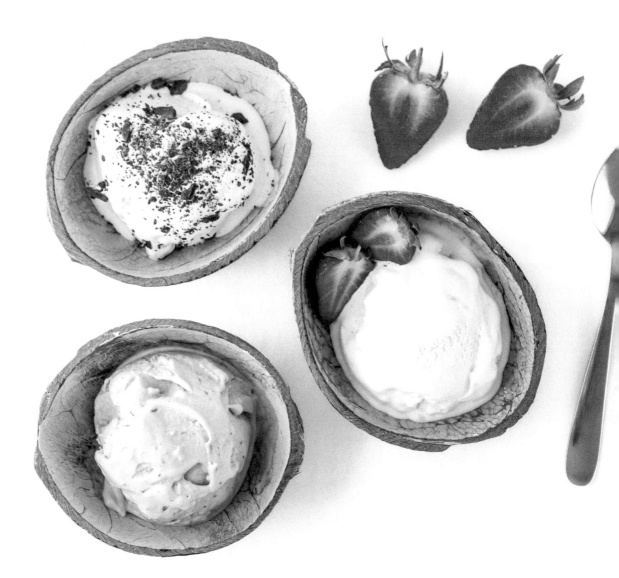

until firm, stirring every 30 minutes for the first 2 hours, then every 60 to 90 minutes. If you want to add mix-ins, stir them in after freezing the ice cream for about 1 hour. If adding berries, puree them in a blender before adding to the ice cream.

6. Store in an airtight container in the freezer for up to 3 months.

KETO CUSTARD

SERVES: 6
PREP TIME: 10 minutes, plus at least 2 hours to chill
COOK TIME: 15 minutes

Nothing beats a good custard. This keto custard is delicious on its own, served with berries, or as a side to a keto pie or cake, like the rhubarb crumble coming up next.

2 cups heavy cream

1 vanilla bean

Pinch of salt

6 large egg yolks

2 tablespoons erythritol

1. Pour the cream into a medium saucepan and start heating over medium heat.

2. Meanwhile, cut the vanilla bean in half lengthwise and scrape out the seeds.

3. Add the vanilla bean pod and seeds to the cream, along with the salt. Heat until just boiling, stirring occasionally, then remove the pan from the heat.

4. In a medium heatproof bowl, whisk together the egg yolks and erythritol until pale.

5. Gradually pour the hot cream mixture into the egg mixture, whisking continuously.

6. Return the mixture to the pan and cook over medium-low heat, whisking constantly, until it thickens. When sufficiently thickened, it will coat the back of a spoon.

7. Once the custard has thickened, remove the vanilla bean. Transfer the custard to a clean heatproof bowl and place in an ice bath. Allow to cool to room temperature, then place plastic wrap directly on top of the custard so it completely covers the surface. This will prevent a skin from forming. Place the bowl in the fridge to chill for 2 to 4 hours before serving.

8. Store in an airtight container in the fridge for up to 4 days.

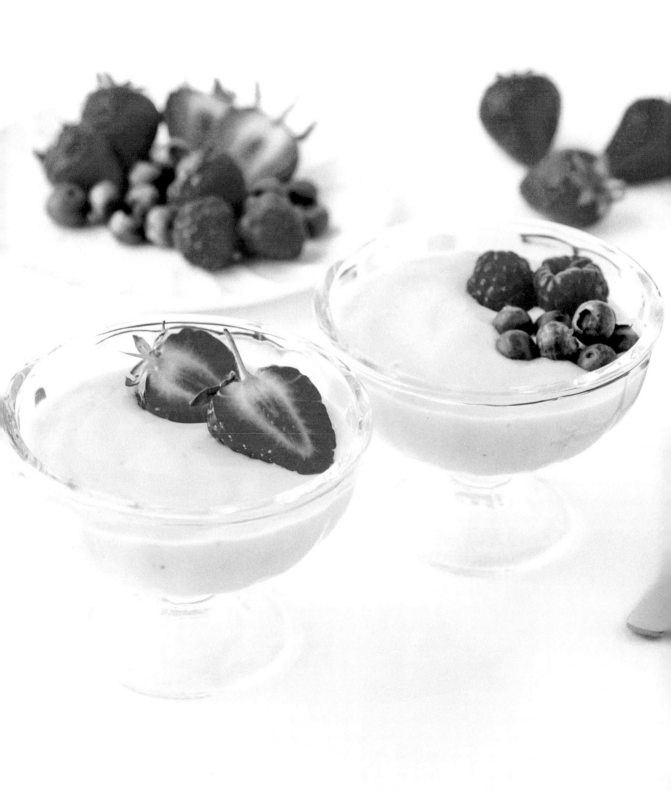

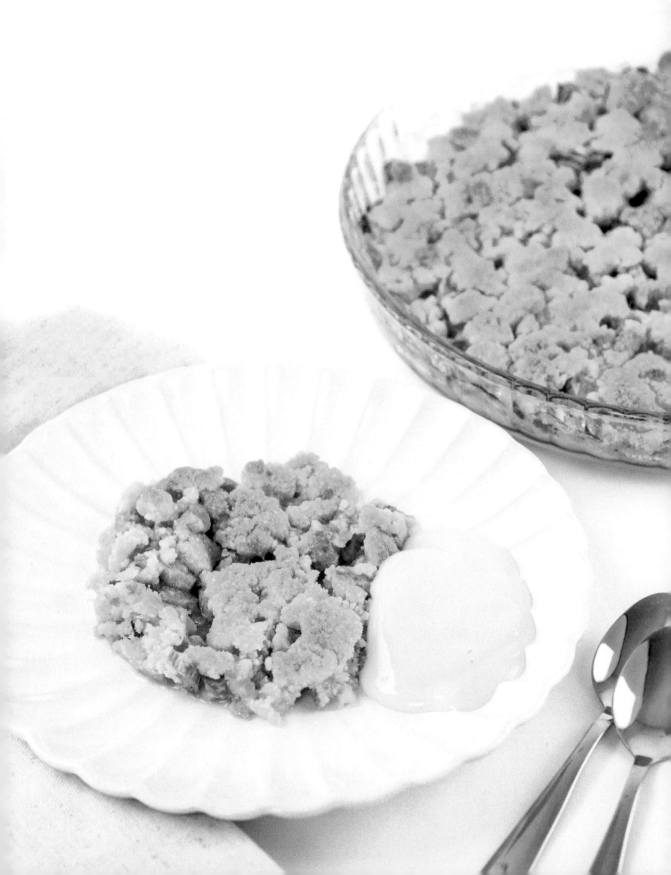

RHUBARB CRUMBLE

SERVES: 8
PREP TIME: 10 minutes
COOK TIME: 30 minutes

Rhubarb is a summer staple in Sweden (where I'm from), and I make this crumble often when rhubarb is in season. This keto-friendly version is just as delicious as the traditional version! It uses almond and coconut flours instead of wheat flour and erythritol instead of sugar. If you want some variety, this crumble recipe works great with blueberries, raspberries, or strawberries as well. In Sweden, fruit crumbles are traditionally served with custard (see page 224), but it also tastes great with ice cream (see page 222).

12 ounces rhubarb

3 to 4 tablespoons erythritol, divided

1 teaspoon xanthan gum

7 tablespoons salted butter, room temperature

¾ cup blanched almond flour

¼ cup coconut flour

1 teaspoon vanilla extract

1 batch Keto Custard (page 224), for serving (optional)

SPECIAL EQUIPMENT (optional):

10-inch ceramic or glass tart pan

1. Preheat the oven to 350°F.

2. Peel the rhubarb and cut it into coins. Transfer to a bowl and mix with 1 tablespoon of the erythritol and the xanthan gum.

3. Using your hands, combine the butter, almond flour, coconut flour, vanilla extract, and remaining 2 to 3 tablespoons of erythritol into a coarse dough. (Note: If you enjoy the tartness of rhubarb, like I do, 2 tablespoons of erythritol will be sufficient; if you find it too tart, go for the full 3 tablespoons.)

4. Cover the bottom of the tart pan with the rhubarb (if you do not have a tart pan, a pie dish will work just as well), then sprinkle the crumble dough on top of the rhubarb. The crumble should roughly cover the whole tart pan, leaving a few gaps.

5. Bake until golden, about 30 minutes.

6. Serve warm, on its own or with custard. Store in the fridge for up to 4 days. Leftovers can be enjoyed cold or reheated in the oven or microwave.

BLUEBERRY PANCAKES

MAKES 8 to 10 small pancakes
(2 per serving)
PREP TIME: 10 minutes
COOK TIME: 30 minutes

Is there anything better than blueberry pancakes? Sure, you can break your fast with these on the weekend, but why not try them for dessert? The French do crêpes for dessert, so you can do pancakes!

3 cups full-fat cottage cheese

4 large eggs

½ cup plus 2 tablespoons psyllium husks

1 teaspoon vanilla extract

Pinch of salt

Salted butter, for the pan

1 cup blueberries, plus more for serving

Whipped cream, for serving (optional)

1. Mix together the cottage cheese, eggs, psyllium husks, vanilla extract, and salt with a wooden spoon. The mixture will be quite thick, more like a dough than a batter. Because it is so thick, you will shape it into pancakes before cooking.

2. Heat a large skillet over medium-low heat. Drop in about ½ tablespoon of butter and allow it to melt.

3. Using your hands, shape a spoonful of the mixture into palm-sized pancakes about ½ inch thick. Place each pancake in the frying pan right away, leaving space between them for flipping.

4. Immediately top the pancakes with blueberries and cook until golden brown on both sides, about 3 minutes total, flipping halfway through.

5. Repeat steps 3 and 4 with the rest of the batter, adding more butter to the pan between batches.

6. Serve with extra blueberries and/or whipped cream.

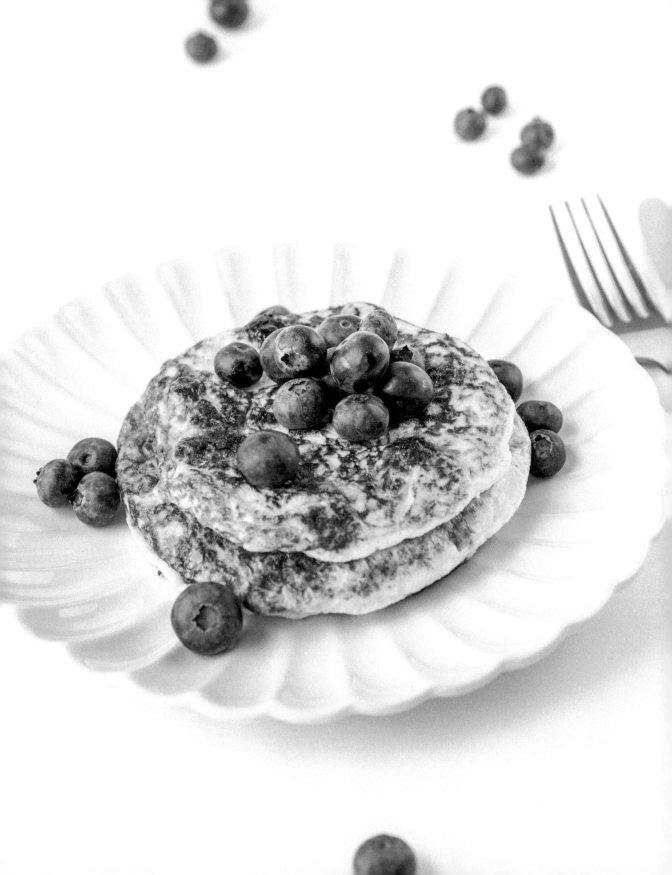

ACKNOWLEDGMENTS

First of all, I want to thank my wonderful husband, Martin, for his unwavering commitment to his vow to always support my dreams and for shooting the cover of this book. I want to thank my mom, Linda; my brother, Johan; my stepdad, Glenn; and all the family and friends who have cheered me on and supported me through this writing journey.

Secondly, I would like to thank Victory Belt Publishing for believing in me and for guiding me through the writing process. Thank you to my editor, Charlotte, for all the hours she's put in to make sure my writing is on point, as well as everyone on the VB team who have had a hand in making this book a reality.

And finally, I want to thank all my clients, customers, and loyal followers who have made this dream a reality. Thank you for encouraging me, believing in me, supporting me, and inspiring me with your stories and commitment to bettering yourself and your health.

And a special thank you to my clients Tammy, Frances, Mandy, Erin, Annaliese, and Carly, who shared their success stories in this book.

FREQUENTLY ASKED QUESTIONS

Sometimes you just need a quick answer to a relatively simple question. Here, I've compiled the answers to some of the most common questions people ask me and answers to get you started on your fasting journey.

Q How do I start fasting?

A There is no one-size-fits-all approach here. Some people are comfortable jumping straight into an extended fast, whereas others want to build up their fasting hours—for example, starting with a sixteen-hour fasting window and an eight-hour eating window and then gradually increasing their fasting hours each day. If you're completely new to fasting, I recommend starting with sixteen hours and building up from there.

Q What advice do you have for a beginner?

A Try it out! Fasting can seem daunting in the beginning, but once you've done it a few times, you will build your confidence and fasting muscle. To avoid uncomfortable side effects, you may want to switch to a ketogenic diet a few days before fasting.

Q What can I eat during my fast?

A You can't eat anything while fasting, but during your eating window, you can eat whatever you like, although I recommend following a keto diet for best results.

Q I really don't eat anything? Only water?

A That's right. When you're fasting, you don't eat anything at all. You can only have water, black coffee, and plain tea. On an extended fast (anything three days or longer), you can also have bone broth and unsweetened pickle juice but never have any sweeteners or sugars.

Q How much weight will I lose?

A How much weight you lose depends on how strict you are and which fasting schedule you're following. As a general rule, you'll lose about 1 pound a day on an extended fast and less if you're on an intermittent fasting schedule.

Q How long should I fast?

A Again, this is completely up to you. The one rule is to fast for only as long as you're physically and mentally comfortable.

Q Will I not starve myself? All of my friends say that my organs will fail!

A No. You are not starving yourself as long as you have enough excess body fat on your body. Your body is designed to fast. Encourage your friends to read up about the benefits of fasting.

Q Can I work while fasting?

A Definitely! Just make sure you keep hydrated and stay on top of your electrolytes so you're not fatigued.

Q Will fasting make me lose muscle?

A You generally won't lose muscle unless you don't have any body fat. Most people have enough body fat to survive several days or even weeks of fasting. Never fast if you're underweight or close to being underweight. If you do, you can lose muscle.

Q Do I have to eat keto in between fasts?

A While I recommend a keto diet, you certainly don't have to eat keto to fast. Many people see great benefits from fasting even without a keto diet. Eating a keto diet is a personal preference, but it can help make fasting easier and also accelerate your fat loss.

Q Will my metabolism slow down?

A No. Fasting has actually been shown to speed up metabolism rather than slowing it down.

Q Can I work out while fasting?

A Absolutely! Many people swear by fasted workouts. The key is to listen to your body. If you're feeling weak or dizzy, make sure you hydrate, take your electrolytes, and adjust the workout intensity as needed.

Q Will a protein shake or pre-workout break my fast?

A Yes, protein shakes and pre-workouts will break your fast. If you want a kick of extra energy before your workout, you can drink a cup of black coffee.

Q What can I drink?

A As a general rule, you can have water, black coffee, and plain tea. For extended fasts, there are a few other liquids you can have. Chapter 9 includes an approved list of liquids.

Q Can I have lemon in my water while fasting?

A You can't squeeze lemon juice into your water, but you can drop in a slice of lemon.

Q Will bulletproof coffee (BPC) break my fast?

A If you're fasting for weight loss and on an extended fast, bulletproof coffee is OK. It has minimal impact (read more in the approved fasting liquids section on page 81). If you're fasting for autophagy, BPC will break autophagy. If you're on a shorter fast or intermittent fasting, you can only have water, black coffee, and plain tea.

Q Are drinks with natural or artificial sweeteners allowed?

A No. Any sweeteners, whether they are natural or artificial, will break your fast.

Q Can I drink coconut water while fasting?

A No. Coconut water is high in carbs and will break your fast.

Q Can I have gum while fasting?

A No. Just as you can't have drinks with natural or artificial sweeteners, gum is off the table. The sweeteners in gum risk spiking your insulin and breaking your fast.

Q Can I take vitamins or supplements while fasting?

A You can take vitamins while fasting, but you don't need to. If you do take them, make sure they aren't sweetened or flavored. Vitamins can make some people feel nauseated when taken on an empty stomach, so skip them if they don't make you feel good. Most supplements contain ingredients or fillers that break your fast, so it's better to take them with a meal.

Q Can I take medications while fasting?

A Always take your prescribed medications, and check with your doctor to verify whether you can take your medicines on an empty stomach.

Q How many calories am I allowed on my days off?

A I don't recommend counting calories. Eat until you're satisfied, no more, no less.

Q Can I fast during my period?

A Yes, you can.

Q Can I fast if I'm pregnant or breastfeeding?

A No. Fasting is not recommended during pregnancy or while breastfeeding.

Q Is it normal to feel cold?

A Yes. Fasting can make you feel cold as blood travels to your vital organs.

Q Is insomnia common?

A Yes, insomnia can be common while fasting, but it's not dangerous. It's your body's natural response to having more energy left over because it isn't digesting food. Fasting also increases your alertness. You can take herbal supplements such as melatonin to help with fasting insomnia.

Q What are electrolytes, and how do I get them?

A You need sodium, potassium, and magnesium while fasting. Many health stores sell electrolytes, or you can buy them online. Make sure you choose products that are unsweetened/unflavored or you'll risk breaking your fast.

Q Is pink salt enough for electrolytes?

A No. Pink salt is a great source of sodium, but you also need potassium and magnesium while you're fasting. The easiest way to get all three is by taking an electrolyte supplement.

Q I have a headache. What should I do?

A A headache is usually a sign of low electrolytes. Try placing some pink salt or sea salt under your tongue to help alleviate the headache.

Q Isn't one meal a day (OMAD) just calorie counting?

A No, not at all. With OMAD, you fast for twenty-three or twenty-four hours and then you have a meal. You don't track your calories. You just eat one meal until you're satisfied.

Q Can I taste the food I'm preparing for my family?

A No. Any food will break your fast, no matter how little.

Q I accidentally ate/swallowed something. Did I break my fast?

A Yes, technically you did. But if it was a genuine mistake, it's not worth throwing your progress away. Keep going with your fast as if nothing happened.

Q In what hour does autophagy peak?

A Autophagy is accelerated during fasting and peaks around thirty-six hours. It will continue to remain high for the full duration of your fast.

Q Can I lose weight on OMAD while not eating keto?

A Yes, absolutely! However, that doesn't mean you can eat whatever you want or however much you want. Always stick to a healthy diet, and only eat until satisfied.

Q Is there a tracker app for my fasting?

A Yes, there are many great fasting tracker apps. Two of the most commonly used ones are Easy Fast and Zero. Search your app store.

Q I'm losing my hair. Is this normal?

A Hair loss is rare, but some people experience this side effect of fasting. If you're worried about hair loss, you can take a biotin supplement.

Q Is store-bought bone broth acceptable?

A When you're on an extended fast, you can have bone broth in small amounts as a crutch (as long as you're fasting for weight loss and not autophagy). Homemade bone broth is the best option because store-bought broths often contain carbs and other additives that break your fast. Making your own bone broth is super easy! My bone broth recipe is on page 176.

Q Where can I go for more information about fasting plans and private coaching.

A For fasting plans, private coaching, and other resources, please visit www.emmavancarlen.com.

ENDNOTES

Chapter 1

1. Keys, A., Brožek, J., Henschel, A., Mickelsen, O., and Taylor, H. L., *The Biology of Human Starvation* (2 volumes), University of Minnesota Press, 1950.

2. Kalm, L. M., and Semba, R. D. (2005). They starved so that others be better fed: remembering Ancel Keys and the Minnesota experiment. *The journal of nutrition*, *135*(6), 1347–1352. https://doi.org/10.1093/jn/135.6.1347.

3. Longo, V. D., and Mattson, M. P. (2014). Fasting: molecular mechanisms and clinical applications. *Cell metabolism*, *19*(2), 181–192. https://doi.org/10.1016/j.cmet.2013.12.008.

4. Kersten S. (2023). The impact of fasting on adipose tissue metabolism. *Biochimica et biophysica acta. Molecular and cell biology of lipids*, 1868(3), 159262. https://doi.org/10.1016/j.bbalip.2022.159262.

5. Stewart, W. K., and Fleming, L. W. (1973). Features of a successful therapeutic fast of 382 days' duration. *Postgraduate medical journal*, *49*(569), 203–209. https://doi.org/10.1136/pgmj.49.569.203.

6. *Guinness Book of World Records*. (1971). Longest Recorded Fast. Guinness World Records.

7. Ooi, T. C., Meramat, A., Rajab, N. F., Shahar, S., Ismail, I. S., Azam, A. A., and Sharif, R. (2020). Intermittent fasting enhanced the cognitive function in older adults with mild cognitive impairment by inducing biochemical and metabolic changes: a 3-year progressive study. *Nutrients*, *12*(9), 2644. https://doi.org/10.3390/nu12092644.

8. Dias, G. P., Murphy, T., Stangl, D., et al. (2021). Intermittent fasting enhances long-term memory consolidation, adult hippocampal neurogenesis, and expression of longevity gene Klotho. *Molecular psychiatry*, *26*(11), 6365-6379. https://doi.org/10.1038/s41380-021-01102-4; Kim, C., Pinto, A. M., Bordoli, C., Buckner, et al. (2020). Energy restriction enhances adult hippocampal neurogenesis-associated memory after four weeks in an adult human population with central obesity; a randomized controlled trial. *Nutrients*, *12*(3), 638. https://doi.org/10.3390/nu12030638.

9. Akan, M., Unal, S., Gonenir Erbay, L., and Taskapan, M. C. (2023). The effect of Ramadan fasting on mental health and some hormonal levels in healthy males. *The Egyptian journal of neurology, psychiatry and neurosurgery*, *59*(1), 20. https://doi.org/10.1186/s41983-023-00623-9.

10. Müller, H., de Toledo, F. W., and Resch, K. L. (2001). Fasting followed by vegetarian diet in patients with rheumatoid arthritis: a systematic review. *Scandinavian journal of rheumatology*, *30*(1), 1–10. https://doi.org/10.1080/030097401750065256.

11. Johnson, J. B., Summer, W., Cutler, R. G., et al. (2007). Alternate day calorie restriction improves clinical findings and reduces markers of oxidative stress and inflammation in overweight adults with moderate asthma. *Free radical biology and medicine*, *42*(5), 665–674. https://doi.org/10.1016/j.freeradbiomed.2006.12.005.

12. Moro, T., Tinsley, G., Bianco, A., et al. (2016). Effects of eight weeks of time-restricted feeding (16/8) on basal metabolism, maximal strength, body composition, inflammation, and cardiovascular risk factors in resistance-trained males. *Journal of translational medicine*, *14*(1), 290. https://doi.org/10.1186/s12967-016-1044-0; Trepanowski, J. F., Kroeger, C. M., Barnosky, A., et al. (2017). Effect of alternate-day fasting on weight loss, weight maintenance, and cardioprotection among metabolically healthy obese adults: a randomized clinical trial. *JAMA internal medicine*, *177*(7), 930–938. https://doi.org/10.1001/jamainternmed.2017.0936.

13. Zarrinpar, A., Chaix, A., Yooseph, S., and Panda, S. (2014). Diet and feeding pattern affect the diurnal dynamics of the gut microbiome. *Cell metabolism, 20*(6), 1006–1017. https://doi.org/10.1016/j.cmet.2014.11.008.

14. Bosy-Westphal, A., Kossel, E., Goele, K., et al. (2009). Contribution of individual organ mass loss to weight loss-associated decline in resting energy expenditure. *The American journal of clinical nutrition, 90*(4), 993–1001. https://doi.org/10.3945/ajcn.2008.27402.

15. Andriessen, C., Doligkeit, D., Moonen-Kornips, E., Mensink, M., Hesselink, M. K. C., Hoeks, J., and Schrauwen, P. (2023). The impact of prolonged fasting on 24h energy metabolism and its 24h rhythmicity in healthy, lean males: a randomized cross-over trial. *Clinical nutrition* (Edinburgh, Scotland), *42*(12), 2353–2362. https://doi.org/10.1016/j.clnu.2023.10.010.

Chapter 2

1. Stratton, M. T., Tinsley, G. M., Alesi, M. G., et al. (2020). Four weeks of time-restricted feeding combined with resistance training does not differentially influence measures of body composition, muscle performance, resting energy expenditure, and blood biomarkers. *Nutrients, 12*(4), 1126. https://doi.org/10.3390/nu12041126; Moro, T., Tinsley, G., Bianco, A., et al. (2016). Effects of eight weeks of time-restricted feeding (16/8) on basal metabolism, maximal strength, body composition, inflammation, and cardiovascular risk factors in resistance-trained males. *Journal of translational medicine, 14*(1), 290. https://doi.org/10.1186/s12967-016-1044-0; Gabel, K., Hoddy, K. K., Haggerty, N., et al. (2018). Effects of 8-hour time restricted feeding on body weight and metabolic disease risk factors in obese adults: A pilot study. *Nutrition and healthy aging, 4*(4), 345–353. https://doi.org/10.3233/NHA-170036.

2. Trepanowski, J. F., Kroeger, C. M., Barnosky, A., et al. (2017). Effects of alternate-day fasting on weight loss, weight maintenance, and cardioprotection among metabolically healthy obese adults: a randomized clinical trial. *JAMA internal medicine, 177*(7), 930–938. https://doi.org/10.1001/jamainternmed.2017.0936; Eshghinia, S., and Mohammadzadeh, F. (2013). The effects of modified alternate-day fasting diet on weight loss and CAD risk factors in overweight and obese women. *Journal of diabetes and metabolic disorders, 12*(1), 4. https://doi.org/10.1186/2251-6581-12-4.

3. Cui Y, Cai T, Zhou Z, et al. Health effects of alternate-day fasting in adults: a systematic review and meta-analysis. (2020). *Frontiers in nutrition,* Nov 24(7):586036. https://doi.org/10.3389/fnut.2020.586036; Goodrick, C. L., Ingram, D. K., Reynolds, M. A., Freeman, J. R., and Cider, N. L. (1982). Effects of intermittent feeding upon growth and life span in rats. *Gerontology, 28*(4), 233–241. https://doi.org/10.1159/000212538.

4. Varady, K. A., Bhutani, S., Klempel, M. C., and Kroeger, C. M. (2011). Comparison of effects of diet versus exercise weight loss regimens on LDL and HDL particle size in obese adults. *Lipids in health and disease, 10*, 119. https://doi.org/10.1186/1476-511X-10-119.

5. Choi, I. Y., Lee, C., and Longo, V. D. (2017). Nutrition and fasting mimicking diets in the prevention and treatment of autoimmune diseases and immunosenescence. *Molecular and cellular endocrinology, 455*, 4–12. https://doi.org/10.1016/j.mce.2017.01.042.

6. Gudden, J., Arias Vasquez, A., and Bloemendaal, M. (2021). The effects of intermittent fasting on brain and cognitive function. *Nutrients, 13*(9), 3166. https://doi.org/10.3390/nu13093166.

7. Jackson, I. M., McKiddie, M. T., and Buchanan, K. D. (1969). Effect of fasting on glucose and insulin metabolism of obese patients. *Lancet.* 1(7589), 285–287. https://doi.org/10.1016/S0140-6736(69)91039-3; Brandhorst, S., Choi, I. Y., Wei, M., et al. (2015). A periodic diet that mimics fasting promotes multi-system regeneration, enhanced cognitive performance, and healthspan. *Cell metabolism, 22*(1), 86–99. https://doi.org/10.1016/j.cmet.2015.05.012.

8. Longo, V. D., and Mattson, M. P. (2014). Fasting: molecular mechanisms and clinical applications. *Cell metabolism*, 19(2), 181–192. https://doi.org/10.1016/j.cmet.2013.12.008

9. Hartman, M. L., Veldhuis, J. D., Johnson, M. L., Lee, M. M., Alberti, K. G., Samojlik, E., and Thorner, M. O. (1992). Augmented growth hormone (GH) secretory burst frequency and amplitude mediate enhanced GH secretion during a two-day fast in normal men. *The journal of clinical endocrinology and metabolism*, 74(4), 757–765. https://doi.org/10.1210/jcem.74.4.1548337; see note 8 above.

10. Ezpeleta, M., Cienfuegos, S., Lin, S., Pavlou, V., Gabel, K., and Varady, K. A. (2023). Efficacy and safety of prolonged water fasting: a narrative review of human trials. *Nutrition reviews*, 82(5), 664–675. https://doi.org/10.1093/nutrit/nuad081.

11. Hallberg, S. J., McKenzie, A. L., Williams, P. T., et al. (2018). Effectiveness and safety of a novel care model for the management of type 2 diabetes at 1 year: an open-label, non-randomized, controlled study. *Diabetes therapy : research, treatment and education of diabetes and related disorders*, 9(2), 583–612. https://doi.org/10.1007/s13300-018-0373-9.

12. Levine, B., and Kroemer, G. (2008). Autophagy in the pathogenesis of disease. *Cell*, 132(1), 27–42. https://doi.org/10.1016/j.cell.2007.12.018.

13. See note 11 above.

14. Hartman, M. L., Veldhuis, J. D., Johnson, M. L., Lee, M. M., Alberti, K. G., Samojlik, E., and Thorner, M. O. (1992). Augmented growth hormone (GH) secretory burst frequency and amplitude mediate enhanced GH secretion during a two-day fast in normal men. *The journal of clinical endocrinology and metabolism*, 74(4), 757–765. https://doi.org/10.1210/jcem.74.4.1548337.

Chapter 3

1. Brillat-Savarin, J. A. (1825). *The Physiology of Taste*. (Trans. by M.K.F. Fisher, 1949). Dover Publications.

2. Banting, W. (1863). *Letter on Corpulence, Addressed to the Public*. Harrison.

3. Shai, I., Schwarzfuchs, D., Henkin, Y., et al. (2008). Weight loss with a low-carbohydrate, Mediterranean, or low-fat diet. *The New England journal of medicine*, 359(3), 229–241. https://doi.org/10.1056/NEJMoa0708681.

4. Statista. Life expectancy (from birth) in the United States, from 1860 to 2020. Accessed May 21, 2024. https://www.statista.com/statistics/1040079/life-expectancy-united-states-all-time/.

5. Martin, S. S. et al. on behalf of the American Heart Association Council on Epidemiology and Prevention Statistics Committee and Stroke Statistics Subcommittee. Heart disease and stroke statistics: a report of US and global data from the American Heart Association, Published online January 24, 2024, https://doi.org/10.1161/CIR.0000000000001209.

6. U.S. Senate Select Committee on Nutrition and Human Needs, Dietary goals for the United States, 2nd ed. (Washington, DC: US Government Printing Office, December 1977).

7. Fryar, C. D., Carroll, M. D., and Afful, J. (2020). Prevalence of overweight, obesity, and severe obesity among adults aged 20 and over: United States, 1960–1962 through 2017–2018. NCHS Health E-Stats. https://www.cdc.gov/nchs/data/hestat/obesity-adult-17-18/overweight-obesity-adults-H.pdf.

8. Melanson, K. J., Angelopoulos, T. J., Nguyen, V. T., et al. (2006). Consumption of whole-grain cereals during weight loss: effects on dietary quality, dietary fiber, magnesium, vitamin

B-6, and obesity. *Journal of the American Dietetic Association, 106*(9), 1380–1390. https://doi.org/10.1016/j.jada.2006.06.003.

9. Lustig, R. H. (2013). *Fat Chance: Beating the Odds Against Sugar, Processed Food, Obesity, and Disease.* Hudson Street Press.

10. Mozaffarian, D., Benjamin, E. J., Go, A. S., et al. Heart disease and stroke statistics–2016 update: a report from the American Heart Association. *Circulation, 133*(4), e38–e360. https://doi.org/10.1161/CIR.0000000000000350.

11. Yudkin, J. (1972). *Pure, White and Deadly: How Sugar is Killing Us.* Penguin Books.

12. Piernas, C., and Popkin, B. M. (2010). Snacking increased among U.S. adults between 1977 and 2006. *The journal of nutrition, 140*(2), 325–332. https://doi.org/10.3945/jn.109.112763.

13. U.S. Department of Agriculture, Agricultural Research Service. 2018. Nutrient intakes from food and beverages: mean amounts consumed per individual, by gender and age. *What We Eat in America.* NHANES 2015-2018.

14. Gearhardt, A., Singer, D., Kirch, M., et al. *Addiction to highly processed food among older adults.* University of Michigan National Poll on Healthy Aging. January/February 2023. Accessed on June 1, 2024. https://dx.doi.org/10.7302/6792.

15. Hruby, A., and Hu, F. B. (2015). The epidemiology of obesity: a big picture. *PharmacoEconomics, 33*(7), 673–689. https://doi.org/10.1007/s40273-014-0243-x.

16. Christakis, N. A., and Fowler, J. H. (2007). The spread of obesity in a large social network over 32 years. *The New England journal of medicine, 357*(4), 370–379. https://doi.org/10.1056/NEJMsa066082.

17. Campbell, M. C., and Mohr, G. S. (2011). Seeing is eating: how and when activation of a negative stereotype increases stereotype-conducive behavior. *Journal of consumer research, 38*(3), 431–444. https://doi.org/10.1086/659754.

Chapter 4

1. Wadden, T. A., Sternberg, J. A., Letizia, K. A., Stunkard, A. J., and Foster G.D. (1989). Treatment of obesity by very low calorie diet, behavior therapy, and their combination: a five-year perspective. *International journal of obesity. 13*(Suppl 2), 39-46. PMID: 2613427.

2. Sumithran, P., Prendergast, L. A., Delbridge, E., Purcell, K., Shulkes, A., Kriketos, A., and Proietto, J. (2011). Long-term persistence of hormonal adaptations to weight loss. *The New England journal of medicine, 365*(17), 1597–1604. https://doi.org/10.1056/NEJMoa1105816.

3. Harvie, M. N., Pegington, M., Mattson, M. P., et al. (2011). The effects of intermittent or continuous energy restriction on weight loss and metabolic disease risk markers: a randomized trial in young overweight women. *International journal of obesity* (2005), *35*(5), 714–727. https://doi.org/10.1038/ijo.2010.171; Patterson, R. E., Laughlin, G. A., LaCroix, A. Z., et al. (2015). Intermittent fasting and human metabolic health. *Journal of the academy of nutrition and dietetics, 115*(8), 1203–1212. https://doi.org/10.1016/j.jand.2015.02.018.

4. Heilbronn, L. K., Smith, S. R., Martin, C. K., Anton, S. D., and Ravussin, E. (2005). Alternate-day fasting in nonobese subjects: effects on body weight, body composition, and energy metabolism. *The American journal of clinical nutrition, 81*(1), 69–73. https://doi.org/10.1093/ajcn/81.1.69.

5. Ho, K. Y., Veldhuis, J. D., Johnson, M. L., Furlanetto, R., Evans, W. S., Alberti, K. G., and Thorner, M. O. (1988). Fasting enhances growth hormone secretion and amplifies the complex rhythms of growth hormone secretion in man. *The journal of clinical investigation, 81*(4), 968–975. https://doi.org/10.1172/JCI113450.

6. Natalucci, G., Riedl, S., Gleiss, A., Zidek, T., and Frisch, H. (2005). Spontaneous 24-h ghrelin secretion pattern in fasting subjects: maintenance of a meal-related pattern. *European journal of endocrinology*, *152*(6), 845–850. https://doi.org/10.1530/eje.1.01919.

7. Zauner, C., Schneeweiss, B., Kranz, A., et al. (2000). Resting energy expenditure in short-term starvation is increased as a result of an increase in serum norepinephrine. *The American journal of clinical nutrition*, *71*(6), 1511–1515. https://doi.org/10.1093/ajcn/71.6.1511.

8. Cummings, D. E., Frayo, R. S., Marmonier, C., Aubert, R., and Chapelot, D. (2004). Plasma ghrelin levels and hunger scores in humans initiating meals voluntarily without time- and food-related cues. *American journal of physiology. Endocrinology and metabolism*, *287*(2), E297–E304. https://doi.org/10.1152/ajpendo.00582.2003.

9. Cahill G. F., Jr (2006). Fuel metabolism in starvation. *Annual review of nutrition*, *26*, 1–22. https://doi.org/10.1146/annurev.nutr.26.061505.111258.

10. Alhamdan, B. A., Garcia-Alvarez, A., Alzahrnai, A. H., et al. (2016). Alternate-day versus daily energy restriction diets: which is more effective for weight loss? A systematic review and meta-analysis. *Obesity science and practice*, *2*(3), 293–302. https://doi.org/10.1002/osp4.52.

11. Rosenbaum, M., and Leibel, R. L. (2010). Adaptive thermogenesis in humans. *International journal of obesity* (2005), *34* (Suppl 1), S47–S55. https://doi.org/10.1038/ijo.2010.184.

12. See note 2 above.

13. Egan, A. M., and Collins, A. L. (2022). Dynamic changes in energy expenditure in response to underfeeding: a review. *PNS: the proceedings of the Nutrition Society*, *81*(2), 199–212. https://doi.org/10.1017/S0029665121003669.

14. Epel, E., Lapidus, R., McEwen, B., and Brownell, K. (2001). Stress may add bite to appetite in women: a laboratory study of stress-induced cortisol and eating behavior. *Psychoneuroendocrinology*, *26*(1), 37–49. https://doi.org/10.1016/s0306-4530(00)00035-4.

15. Steptoe, A., Kunz-Ebrecht, S. R., Brydon, L., and Wardle, J. (2004). Central adiposity and cortisol responses to waking in middle-aged men and women. *International journal of obesity*. *28*(9),1168–1173. https://doi.org/10.1038/sj.ijo.0802715.

16. Ainsworth, B. E., Haskell, W. L., Herrmann, S. D., et al. (2011). 2011 compendium of physical activities: a second update of codes and MET values. *Medicine and science in sports and exercise*, *43*(8), 1575–1581. https://doi.org/10.1249/MSS.0b013e31821ece12.

17. Swift, D. L., McGee, J. E., Earnest, C. P., Carlisle, E., Nygard, M., and Johannsen, N. M. (2018). The effects of exercise and physical activity on weight loss and maintenance. *Progress in cardiovascular diseases*, *61*(2), 206–213. https://doi.org/10.1016/j.pcad.2018.07.014.

18. Johns, D. J., Hartmann-Boyce, J., Jebb, S. A., Aveyard, P., and Behavioural Weight Management Review Group. (2014). Diet or exercise interventions vs combined behavioral weight management programs: a systematic review and meta-analysis of direct comparisons. *Journal of the Academy of Nutrition and Dietetics*, *114*(10), 1557–1568. https://doi.org/10.1016/j.jand.2014.07.005.

19. Jafari, A., Maghsoud, P., Azarbayejani, M. A., Homai, H. M. (2017). Effect of resistance training on appetite regulation and level of related peptidesin sedentary healthy men. *Medical laboratory journal*, *11*(4), 24–29. https://doi.org/ 10.18869/acadpub.mlj.11.4.24.

20. Callahan, M. (2015). The brutal secrets behind 'The Biggest Loser.' *New York Post* website, accessed May 23, 2024. https://nypost.com/2015/01/18/contestant-reveals-the-brutal-secrets-of-the-biggest-loser/.

21. Fothergill, E., Guo, J., Howard, L., et al. (2016). Persistent metabolic adaptation 6 years after "The Biggest Loser" competition. *Obesity* (Silver Spring, Md.), *24*(8), 1612–1619. https://doi.org/10.1002/oby.21538.

22. Dulloo, A. G., Jacquet, J., Montani, J. P., and Schutz, Y. (2012). Adaptive thermogenesis in human body weight regulation: more of a concept than a measurable entity? *Obesity reviews : an official journal of the International Association for the Study of Obesity, 13* (Suppl 2), 105–121. https://doi.org/10.1111/j.1467-789X.2012.01041.x.

23. See note 21 above.

24. See note 20 above.

25. See note 21 above.

26. Kolata, G. (2016). After 'The Biggest Loser,' their bodies fought to regain weight. *New York Times* website, accessed May 23, 2024. https://www.nytimes.com/2016/05/02/health/biggest-loser-weight-loss.html.

27. Keys, A., Brozek, J., Henschel, A., Mickelsen, O., and Taylor, H. L., *The Biology of Human Starvation* (2 volumes), University of Minnesota Press, 1950.

28. See note 20 above; Katz, N. (2010). "Biggest Loser" contestant Kai Hibbard slams reality show, gained weight back. CBS News website, accessed May 23, 2024. https://www.cbsnews.com/news/biggest-loser-contestant-kai-hibbard-slams-reality-show-gained-weight-back/.

29. See note 20 above.

Chapter 5

1. Kiecolt-Glaser, J. K., Habash, D. L., Fagundes, C. P., Andridge, R., Peng, J., Malarkey, W. B., and Belury, M. A. (2015). Daily stressors, past depression, and metabolic responses to high-fat meals: a novel path to obesity. *Biological psychiatry, 77*(7), 653–660. https://doi.org/10.1016/j.biopsych.2014.05.018.

2. Allard, C., Doyon, M., Brown, C., Carpentier, A. C., Langlois, M. F., and Hivert, M. F. (2013). Lower leptin levels are associated with higher risk of weight gain over 2 years in healthy young adults. *Applied physiology, nutrition, and metabolism = Physiologie appliquee, nutrition et metabolisme, 38*(3), 280–285. https://doi.org/10.1139/apnm-2012-0225.

3. Considine, R. V., Sinha, M. K., Heiman, M. L., et al. (1996). Serum immunoreactive-leptin concentrations in normal-weight and obese humans. *The New England journal of medicine, 334*(5), 292–295. https://doi.org/10.1056/NEJM199602013340503.

4. Gruzdeva, O., Borodkina, D., Uchasova, E., Dyleva, Y., and Barbarash, O. (2019). Leptin resistance: underlying mechanisms and diagnosis. *Diabetes, metabolic syndrome and obesity : targets and therapy, 12*, 191–198. https://doi.org/10.2147/DMSO.S182406.

5. Pérez-Pérez, A., Sánchez-Jiménez, F., Vilariño-García, T., and Sánchez-Margalet, V. (2020). Role of leptin in inflammation and vice versa. *International journal of molecular sciences, 21*(16), 5887. https://doi.org/10.3390/ijms21165887.

6. Briscoe, C. P., Hanif, S., Arch, J. R. S., and Tadayyon, M. (2001). Fatty acids inhibit leptin signalling in BRIN-BD11 insulinoma cells. J*ournal of molecular endocrinology, 26*(2), 145. https://doi.org/10.1677/jme.0.0260145.

7. See note 4 above.

8. Perrigue, M. M., Drewnowski, A., Wang, C. Y., and Neuhouser, M. L. (2016). Higher eating frequency does not decrease appetite in healthy adults. *The journal of nutrition, 146*(1), 59–64. https://doi.org/10.3945/jn.115.216978.

9. Leidy, H. J., Tang, M., Armstrong, C. L., Martin, C. B., and Campbell, W. W. (2011). The effects of consuming frequent, higher protein meals on appetite and satiety during weight loss in overweight/obese men. *Obesity* (Silver Spring, Md.), *19*(4), 818–824. https://doi.org/10.1038/oby.2010.203.

10. Natalucci, G., Riedl, S., Gleiss, A., Zidek, T., and Frisch, H. (2005). Spontaneous 24-h ghrelin secretion pattern in fasting subjects: maintenance of a meal-related pattern. *European journal of endocrinology*, *152*(6), 845–850. https://doi.org/10.1530/eje.1.01919.

11. Espelund, U., Hansen, T. K., Højlund, K., et al. (2005). Fasting unmasks a strong inverse association between ghrelin and cortisol in serum: studies in obese and normal-weight subjects. *The journal of clinical endocrinology and metabolism*, *90*(2), 741–746. https://doi.org/10.1210/jc.2004-0604.

12. Goldstein D. S. (2010). Adrenal responses to stress. *Cellular and molecular neurobiology*, *30*(8), 1433–1440. https://doi.org/10.1007/s10571-010-9606-9.

13. See note 1 above.

14. Spiegel, K., Leproult, R., and Van Cauter, E. (1999). Impact of sleep debt on metabolic and endocrine function. *Lancet* (London, England), *354*(9188), 1435–1439. https://doi.org/10.1016/S0140-6736(99)01376-8.

15. Cahill G. F., Jr (2006). Fuel metabolism in starvation. *Annual review of nutrition*, *26*, 1–22. https://doi.org/10.1146/annurev.nutr.26.061505.111258.

16. Patterson, R. E., Laughlin, G. A., LaCroix, A. Z., et al. (2015). Intermittent fasting and human metabolic health. *Journal of the Academy of Nutrition and Dietetics*, *115*(8), 1203–1212. https://doi.org/10.1016/j.jand.2015.02.018.

17. Harvie, M. N., Pegington, M., Mattson, M. P., et al. (2011). The effects of intermittent or continuous energy restriction on weight loss and metabolic disease risk markers: a randomized trial in young overweight women. *International journal of obesity* (2005), *35*(5), 714–727. https://doi.org/10.1038/ijo.2010.171.

Chapter 6

1. Redman, L. M., Heilbronn, L. K., Martin, C. K., et al. (2009). Metabolic and behavioral compensations in response to caloric restriction: implications for the maintenance of weight loss. *PloS one*, *4*(2), e4377. https://doi.org/10.1371/journal.pone.0004377.

2. Zauner, C., Schneeweiss, B., Kranz, A., et al. (2000). Resting energy expenditure in short-term starvation is increased as a result of an increase in serum norepinephrine. *The American journal of clinical nutrition*, *71*(6), 1511–1515. https://doi.org/10.1093/ajcn/71.6.1511; Mansell, P. I., Fellows, I. W., and Macdonald, I. A. (1990). Enhanced thermogenic response to epinephrine after 48-h starvation in humans. *The American journal of physiology*, *258*(1 Pt 2), R87–R93. https://doi.org/10.1152/ajpregu.1990.258.1.R87.

3. Patel, J. N., Coppack, S. W., Goldstein, D. S., Miles, J. M., and Eisenhofer, G. (2002). Norepinephrine spillover from human adipose tissue before and after a 72-hour fast. *The journal of clinical endocrinology and metabolism*, *87*(7), 3373–3377. https://doi.org/10.1210/jcem.87.7.8695; see note 2 above.

4. Hartman, M. L., Veldhuis, J. D., Johnson, M. L., Lee, M. M., Alberti, K. G., Samojlik, E., and Thorner, M. O. (1992). Augmented growth hormone (GH) secretory burst frequency and amplitude mediate enhanced GH secretion during a two-day fast in normal men. *The journal of clinical endocrinology and metabolism*, *74*(4), 757–765. https://doi.org/10.1210/jcem.74.4.1548337.

5. Rosenbaum, M., and Leibel, R. L. Adaptive thermogenesis in humans. (2010). *International journal of obesity* (London). *34*(Suppl 1), S47–55. https://doi.org/10.1038/ijo.2010.184.

6. Ishii, S., Osaki, N., and Shimotoyodome, A. (2016). The effects of a hypocaloric diet on diet-induced thermogenesis and blood hormone response in healthy male adults: a pilot study.

Journal of nutritional science and vitaminology, 62(1), 40–46. https://doi.org/10.3177/jnsv.62.40; Most, J., and Redman, L. M. (2020). Impact of calorie restriction on energy metabolism in humans. *Experimental gerontology, 133*, 110875. https://doi.org/10.1016/j.exger.2020.110875.

7. Catenacci, V. A., Pan, Z., Ostendorf, D., et al. (2016). A randomized pilot study comparing zero-calorie alternate-day fasting to daily caloric restriction in adults with obesity. *Obesity* (Silver Spring, Md.), *24*(9), 1874–1883. https://doi.org/10.1002/oby.21581.

8. See note 2 above.

9. See note 3 above.

10. Raichle, M. E., and Gusnard, D. A. (2002). Appraising the brain's energy budget. *Proceedings of the National Academy of Sciences of the United States of America, 99*(16), 10237–10239. https://doi.org/10.1073/pnas.172399499.

11. Courchesne-Loyer, A., Croteau, E., Castellano, C. A., St-Pierre, V., Hennebelle, M., and Cunnane, S. C. (2017). Inverse relationship between brain glucose and ketone metabolism in adults during short-term moderate dietary ketosis: A dual tracer quantitative positron emission tomography study. *Journal of cerebral blood flow and metabolism : official journal of the International Society of Cerebral Blood Flow and Metabolism, 37*(7), 2485–2493. https://doi.org/10.1177/0271678X16669366.

12. See note 11 above.

13. White, H., and Venkatesh, B. (2011). Clinical review: ketones and brain injury. *Critical care* (London, England), *15*(2), 219. https://doi.org/10.1186/cc10020.

14. Zhang, X., Yang, S., Chen, J., and Su, Z. (2019). Unraveling the regulation of hepatic gluconeogenesis. *Frontiers in endocrinology, 9*, 802. https://doi.org/10.3389/fendo.2018.00802.

15. Varady, K. A., Bhutani, S., Klempel, M. C., et al. (2013). Alternate day fasting for weight loss in normal weight and overweight subjects: a randomized controlled trial. *Nutrition journal, 12*, 1-8. https://doi.org/10.1186/1475-2891-12-146.

16. See note 15 above.

17. Stote, K. S., Baer, D. J., Spears, K., et al. (2007). A controlled trial of reduced meal frequency without caloric restriction in healthy, normal-weight, middle-aged adults. *The American journal of clinical nutrition, 85*(4), 981–988. https://doi.org/10.1093/ajcn/85.4.981.

18. Johnstone, A. M., Faber, P., Gibney, E. R., Elia, M., Horgan, G., Golden, B. E., and Stubbs, R. J. (2002). Effect of an acute fast on energy compensation and feeding behaviour in lean men and women. *International journal of obesity and related metabolic disorders : journal of the International Association for the Study of Obesity, 26*(12), 1623–1628. https://doi.org/10.1038/sj.ijo.0802151.

19. Cummings, D. E., Purnell, J. Q., Frayo, R. S., Schmidova, K., Wisse, B. E., and Weigle, D. S. (2001). A preprandial rise in plasma ghrelin levels suggests a role in meal initiation in humans. *Diabetes, 50*(8), 1714–1719. https://doi.org/10.2337/diabetes.50.8.1714.

20. Espelund, U., Hansen, T. K., Højlund, K., et al. (2005). Fasting unmasks a strong inverse association between ghrelin and cortisol in serum: studies in obese and normal-weight subjects. *The journal of clinical endocrinology and metabolism, 90*(2), 741–746. https://doi.org/10.1210/jc.2004-0604.

21. See note 20 above.

22. Natalucci, G., Riedl, S., Gleiss, A., Zidek, T., and Frisch, H. (2005). Spontaneous 24-h ghrelin secretion pattern in fasting subjects: maintenance of a meal-related pattern. *European journal of endocrinology, 152*(6), 845–850. https://doi.org/10.1530/eje.1.01919.

23. Ravussin, E., Beyl, R. A., Poggiogalle, E., Hsia, D. S., and Peterson, C. M. (2019). Early time-restricted feeding reduces appetite and increases fat oxidation but does not affect energy expenditure in humans. *Obesity* (Silver Spring, Md.), *27*(8), 1244–1254. https://doi.org/10.1002/oby.22518.

Chapter 7

1. Sinha, R., Gu, P., Hart, R., and Guarnaccia, J. B. (2019). Food craving, cortisol and ghrelin responses in modeling highly palatable snack intake in the laboratory. *Physiology & behavior*, *208*, 112563. https://doi.org/10.1016/j.physbeh.2019.112563.

Chapter 8

1. Ho, K. Y., Veldhuis, J. D., Johnson, M. L., Furlanetto, R., Evans, W. S., Alberti, K. G., and Thorner, M. O. (1988). Fasting enhances growth hormone secretion and amplifies the complex rhythms of growth hormone secretion in man. *The journal of clinical investigation*, *81*(4), 968–975. https://doi.org/10.1172/JCI113450.

2. Achten, J., and Jeukendrup, A. E. (2004). Optimizing fat oxidation through exercise and diet. *Nutrition* (Burbank, Los Angeles County, Calif.), *20*(7–8), 716–727. https://doi.org/10.1016/j.nut.2004.04.005.

Chapter 10

1. Chevalier, G., Sinatra, S. T., Oschman, J. L., Sokal, K., and Sokal, P. (2012). Earthing: health implications of reconnecting the human body to the Earth's surface electrons. *Journal of environmental and public health*. *2012*, 291541. https://doi.org/10.1155/2012/291541.

2. Lochbaum, M., Sherburn, M., Sisneros, C., Cooper, S., Lane, A. M., and Terry, P. C. (2022). Revisiting the self-confidence and sport performance relationship: a systematic review with meta-analysis. *International journal of environmental research and public health*, *19*(11), 6381. https://doi.org/10.3390/ijerph19116381; Mavros, M. N., Athanasiou, S., Gkegkes, I. D., Polyzos, K. A., Peppas, G., and Falagas, M. E. (2011). Do psychological variables affect early surgical recovery? *PloS one*, *6*(5), e20306. https://doi.org/10.1371/journal.pone.0020306.

3. Brown W. A. (2015). Expectation, the placebo effect and the response to treatment. *Rhode Island medical journal* (2013), *98*(5), 19–21.

4. Hynes, J. and Turner, Z. (2020). Positive visualization and its effects on strength training. *Impulse: the premier undergraduate neuroscience journal*. Transylvania University, Lexington, KY, United States, 40508. https://assets.pubpub.org/k9og4slt/31643844339559.pdf.

5. Ranganathan, V. K., Siemionow, V., Liu, J. Z., Sahgal, V., and Yue, G. H. (2004). From mental power to muscle power—gaining strength by using the mind. *Neuropsychologia*, *42*(7), 944–956. https://doi.org/10.1016/j.neuropsychologia.2003.11.018.

6. Cascio, C. N., O'Donnell, M. B., Tinney, F. J., Lieberman, M. D., Taylor, S. E., Strecher, V. J., and Falk, E. B. (2016). Self-affirmation activates brain systems associated with self-related processing and reward and is reinforced by future orientation. *Social cognitive and affective neuroscience*, *11*(4), 621–629. https://doi.org/10.1093/scan/nsv136.

Chapter 11

1. Morey, J. N., Boggero, I. A., Scott, A. B., and Segerstrom, S. C. (2015). Current directions in stress and human immune function. *Current opinion in psychology, 5*, 13–17. https://doi.org/10.1016/j.copsyc.2015.03.007; Rohleder N. (2014). Stimulation of systemic low-grade inflammation by psychosocial stress. *Psychosomatic medicine, 76*(3), 181–189. https://doi.org/10.1097/PSY.0000000000000049.

2. Finassi, C. M., Calixto, L. A., Segura, W., et al. (2023). Effect of sweetened beverages intake on salivary aspartame, insulin and alpha-amylase levels: A single-blind study. Food research international (Ottawa, Ont.), 173(Pt 2), 113406. https://doi.org/10.1016/j.foodres.2023.113406; Hu, Y., Costenbader, K. H., Gao, X., et al. (2014). Sugar-sweetened soda consumption and risk of developing rheumatoid arthritis in women. The American journal of clinical nutrition, 100(3), 959–967. https://doi.org/10.3945/ajcn.114.086918; Finamor, I. A., Bressan, C. A., Torres-Cuevas, I., et al. (2021). Long-term aspartame administration leads to fibrosis, inflammasome activation, and gluconeogenesis impairment in the liver of mice. Biology, 10(2), 82. https://doi.org/10.3390/biology10020082.

3. Suez, J., Korem, T., Zeevi, D., et al. (2014). Artificial sweeteners induce glucose intolerance by altering the gut microbiota. Nature, 514(7521), 181–186. https://doi.org/10.1038/nature13793; Zhao, M., Chu, J., Feng, S., et al. (2023). Immunological mechanisms of inflammatory diseases caused by gut microbiota dysbiosis: a review. Biomedicine & Pharmacotherapy, 164. https://doi.org/10.1016/j.biopha.2023.114985.

4. Mullington, J. M., Simpson, N. S., Meier-Ewert, H. K., and Haack, M. (2010). Sleep loss and inflammation. Best practice & research. Clinical endocrinology & metabolism, 24(5), 775–784. https://doi.org/10.1016/j.beem.2010.08.014.

5. Quertemont, E., and Didone, V. (2006). Role of acetaldehyde in mediating the pharmacological and behavioral effects of alcohol. Alcohol research & health : the journal of the National Institute on Alcohol Abuse and Alcoholism, 29(4), 258–265; Seitz, H. K., and Becker, P. (2007). Alcohol metabolism and cancer risk. Alcohol research & health : the journal of the National Institute on Alcohol Abuse and Alcoholism, 30(1), 38–47.

6. Chaput J. P. (2014). Sleep patterns, diet quality and energy balance. Physiology & behavior, 134, 86–91. https://doi.org/10.1016/j.physbeh.2013.09.006.

Chapter 12

1. Mehanna, H. M., Moledina, J., and Travis, J. (2008). Refeeding syndrome: what it is, and how to prevent and treat it. BMJ (Clinical research ed.), 336(7659), 1495–1498. https://doi.org/10.1136/bmj.a301.

2. Shukla, A. P., Andono, J., Touhamy, S. H., et al. (2017). Carbohydrate-last meal pattern lowers postprandial glucose and insulin excursions in type 2 diabetes. BMJ open diabetes research & care, 5(1), e000440. https://doi.org/10.1136/bmjdrc-2017-000440.

3. Freitas, D., and Le Feunteun, S., (2018). Acid induced reduction of the glycaemic response to starch-rich foods: the salivary ⍺-amylase inhibition hypothesis. Food & function, 9(10), 5096–5102. https://doi.org/10.1039/c8fo01489b.

4. Stiemsma, L. T., Nakamura, R. E., Nguyen, J. G., and Michels, K. B. (2020). Does consumption of fermented foods modify the human gut microbiota? The journal of nutrition, 150(7), 1680–1692. https://doi.org.10.1093/jn/nxaa077

5. Wastyk, H. C., Fragiadakis, G. K., Perelman, D., et al. (2021). Gut-microbiota-targeted diets modulate human immune status. Cell, 184(16), 4137–4153. https://doi.org/10.1016/j.cell.2021.06.019.

6. Pepino, M. Y., Tiemann, C. D., Patterson, B. W., Wice, B. M., and Klein, S. (2013). Sucralose affects glycemic and hormonal responses to an oral glucose load. *Diabetes care*, *36*(9), 2530–2535. https://doi.org/10.2337/dc12-2221.

7. Mathur, K., Agrawal, R. K., Nagpure, S., and Deshpande, D. (2020). Effect of artificial sweeteners on insulin resistance among type-2 diabetes mellitus patients. *Journal of family medicine and primary care*, *9*(1), 69–71. https://doi.org/10.4103/jfmpc.jfmpc_329_19.

8. Wang, Q. P., Lin, Y. Q., Zhang, L., et al. (2016). Sucralose promotes food intake through NPY and a neuronal fasting response. *Cell metabolism*, *24*(1), 75–90. https://doi.org/10.1016/j.cmet.2016.06.010; see note 7 above.

Chapter 14

1. Tribole, E., and Resch, E. (1995). *Intuitive Eating: A Revolutionary Program that Works*. New York: St. Martin's Press

2. Lappalainen, R., Sjödén, P. O., Hursti, T., and Vesa, V. (1990). Hunger/craving responses and reactivity to food stimuli during fasting and dieting. *International journal of obesity*, *14*(8), 679–688; Espelund, U., Hansen, T. K., Højlund, K., et al. (2005). Fasting unmasks a strong inverse association between ghrelin and cortisol in serum: studies in obese and normal-weight subjects. *The journal of clinical endocrinology and metabolism*, *90*(2), 741–746. https://doi.org/10.1210/jc.2004-0604; Deemer, S. E., Plaisance, E. P., and Martins, C. (2020). Impact of ketosis on appetite regulation-a review. *Nutrition research* (New York, N.Y.), *77*, 1–11. https://doi.org/10.1016/j.nutres.2020.02.010.

FURTHER READING

Ajoolabady et al. "Targeting Autophagy in Neurodegenerative Diseases"

Baker, "Body Weight and the Initiation of Puberty"

Cava et al., "Preserving Healthy Muscle During Weight Loss"

Chaix et al., "Time-Restricted Feeding Is a Preventative and Therapeutic Intervention Against Diverse Nutritional Challenges"

Clapp et al., "Gut Microbiota's Effect on Mental Health"

Colrain et al., "Alcohol and the Sleeping Brain"

Cryan, "Mind-Altering Microorganisms"

de Cabo & Mattson, "Effects of Intermittent Fasting on Health, Aging, and Disease"

Epel et al, "Stress May Add Bite to Appetite in Women"

Field et al., "Acute Alcohol Effects on Inhibitory Control and Implicit Cognition"

Flier, "Obesity Wars: Molecular Progress Confronts an Expanding Epidemic"

Friedman & Halaas, "Leptin and the Regulation of Body Weight in Mammals"

Furmli et al., "Therapeutic Use of Intermittent Fasting for People with Type 2 Diabetes as an Alternative to Insulin"

Goyal et al., "Meditation Programs for Psychological Stress and Well-Being"

Green et al., "Lack of Effect of Short-Term Fasting on Cognitive Function"

Horne et al., "Health Effects of Intermittent Fasting"

Leeuwendaal et al., "Fermented Foods, Health and the Gut Microbiome"

Leibel et al., "Changes in Energy Expenditure Resulting from Altered Body Weight"

Leproult et al., "Role of Sleep and Sleep Loss in Hormonal Release and Metabolism"

Libby, "Inflammation in Atherosclerosis"

Ludwig & Ebbeling, "The Carbohydrate-Insulin Model of Obesity"

Madeo et al., "Essential Role for Autophagy in Life Span Extension"

Martin et al., "The Role of Diet on the Gut Microbiome, Mood and Happiness"

Medzhitov, "Origin and Physiological Roles of Inflammation"

Mizushima & Komatsu, "Autophagy: Renovation of Cells and Tissues"

Myers et al., "Mechanisms of Leptin Action and Leptin Resistance"

NIH National Institute on Aging, *Heart Health and Aging*

Okabayashi et al., "Diagnosis and Management of Insulinoma"

Paoli et al., "The Effects of Ketogenic Diet on Insulin Sensitivity and Weight Loss, Which Came First: The Chicken or the Egg?"

Paoli et al., "A Review of the Therapeutic Uses of Very-Low-Carbohydrate (Ketogenic) Diets"

Patterson & Sears, "Metabolic Effects of Intermittent Fasting"

Reaven, "Banting Lecture 1988. Role of Insulin Resistance in Human Disease"

Rosmond, "Role of Stress in the Pathogenesis of the Metabolic Syndrome"

Russell-Jones & Khan, "Insulin-Associated Weight Gain in Diabetes"

Saltiel & Kahn, "Insulin Signalling and the Regulation of Glucose and Lipid Metabolism"

Schwartz et al., "Central Nervous System Control of Food Intake"

Turicchi et al., "Weekly, Seasonal and Holiday Body Weight Fluctuation Patterns Among Individuals Engaged in a European Multi-Centre Behavioural Weight Loss Maintenance Intervention"

Veldhuis et al., "Endocrine Control of Body Composition in Infancy, Childhood, and Puberty"

Volek & Phinney, "The Art and Science of Low Carbohydrate Performance: A Revolutionary Program to Extend Your Physical and Mental Performance Envelope"

White et al., "Autophagy, Metabolism, and Cancer"

Yau & Potenza, "Stress and Eating Behaviors"

INDEX

Victory Belt Publishing
3145 W Torino Ave.
US-NV, 89118
US
https://www.victorybelt.com
859-663-8017

The authorized representative in the EU for product safety and compliance is

YoBo Graphics Ltd
Boryana Vasileva Yordanova
26 Bulair Str.
ECZ, 4000
BG
yobo@victorybelt.com

ISBN: 9781628605112
Release ID: 150816563